Sleep fo Bab

C000091588

The Nighttime Sleep Solution to Your Infant

Sleeping Problems

Regina Williams

Copyright © 2020 Regina Williams

All rights reserved. No part of this publication may be reproduced, distributed, or transmitted in any form or by any means, including photocopying, recording, or other electronic or mechanical methods, without the prior written permission of the publisher, except in the case of brief quotations embodied in critical reviews and specific other non-commercial uses permitted by copyright law.

978-1-63750-012-5

Published By:

Healthy Lifestyle Books

Website: www.engolee.com/bookdeals

Email: info@engolee.com

Table of Contents

Introduction

Are you nursing a baby and you want to know more about what to expect during the first few years of nursing a baby as either a first time mother or father or already a mother or father, or do you wish to gift book on nursing a baby to new parents?

This is the guide to meet all your need. It's a comprehensive book that talks about the nature of babies.

It could be debilitating if you are exhausted or more during the night to soothe your crying baby, mainly if you had a long day. We'll begin with why a baby isn't sleeping and ways to help her to rest better.

When babies can't rest, they may be experiencing challenges like the common life-long struggle that lots of people have as it pertains right down to bedtime. Many people develop sleeplessness from certain sets off, such as too much caffeine, display screen time too near to the night, or only excess stress.

Babies have their group of sleeplessness sets off that may

keep them from a good evening rest. Being conscious of why your child won't rest, can't sleep, or requires continuous co-sleeping is the first step to resolving those problems.

In this book you will learn sleep program that is strongly suggested if you want assistance in getting the baby to drift off and stay asleep, how to set bed time regimen, ways to turn your child from a crib to toddler bed, common baby sleep myths, how babies adapt to timezone changes, childhood sleep apnea, reasons why your child won't laugh or happy, what to do when your baby sleep with eyes opened, food to avoid and food to eat, and many more!

After reading this book, you would be well equipped with what to expect during the first year of childbirth and nurturing of your baby.

Chapter 1

Factors that Causes Babies' Sleeplessness

1. Over-Stimulation

When the surrounding is too stimulating, your child may have trouble calming down. This may make it hard to access sleep when it is bedtime and might even make your child become hyper-alert, fidgety or even stressed.

Their growing brain can become too overwhelmed by every new signal it gets. Each experience and new feeling is another neuron firing. Many of these thrill their experience in building reliable systems in their brains which is vital for brain development, infants need a rest from this stimulation to be able to process everything. While asleep, the brain does the job of clearing up every one of the structures in the neurons; recollections are processed, encounters are submitted away, and the mind cleans itself up from the waste materials, by-products of the power it used.

Reducing stimulation near to bedtime can help their brain

get into a reasonable condition. The stimulus will come in the proper execution of sounds, speaking, books, toys, fired up televisions or displays, or talking encounters taking a look at them.

2. Too little Routine

Although your pacing babies' day according to her cues, everyone can still reap the benefits of a healthy routine, hence, rather than trying to place her on a good schedule, concentrate on assisting by figuring out how to associate times of your day with certain activities.

Routine helps to create positive targets, it helps the body and brain turn to cues for what's next and the body may then be modified to these targets, planning for another activity. These types of balance are so very important for babies just as a sense of uniformity is beneficial for members of a family.

This also marvellously results in bedtime. As night time approaches, they could commence detecting the cues; the dimming lighting, the quieting of activity and the change of environment might all help signal to their brain that rest is coming.

3. Overtiredness or Nap-Deprived

If you've ever had an evening where you pushed yourself to ultimately stay awake and finally got to bed but found that your brain couldn't decelerate, you've experienced what is referred to as *overtiredness*.

Infants get that too. If indeed they push themselves to remain awake when their body begins giving sleepy indicators, they''ll likely create a habit to do a similar thing when it's time to visit sleep. They'll wake up more, fuss more, and stay away from sleeping. Make an effort to offer your child more naps each day and a consistent bedtime rest.

It may appear just a little counter-intuitive if a baby isn't getting back enough naps, it's much more likely they won't have the ability to decrease for bedtime either. Infants under twelve months typically need to rest every two hours; an infant that is under half a year old only must be awake for one and a half hours before going down for a nap again.

4. Another reason includes a Sore neck or a Hearing Infection

You may know very well what it's preferred to make an effort to sleep with a cold. A sore throat can be agonizing and keep you in a routine of pain that retains you from calming. If your child is getting up suddenly and crying in distress, it might be a sign the baby is distressed by the pain of the ear illness or a sore neck.

While these are typically normal for an infant to experience, it could be hard with their under-developed immune systems to battle off chlamydia. Be sure to take your child to a pediatrician if you believe this is the problem.

Look out for thick yellow release from the nasal area or bloating and puffiness around the nose and eye.

5. Food Allergies or Sensitivities

Using the rise of food sensitivities, it looks like increasingly more children are being identified as having food allergies. Your child may be delicate to a particular food, too.

These sensitivities can irritate the digestive tract and cause general discomfort for your child, and they could feel itchy or have acid reflux disorder that is keeping them up during the night. If your child is showing indications of colic stress or developing unexplained or extreme rashes, food allergies should be contained in your investigation.

You can begin by removing common food allergens to find out if your baby reacts positively. Foods such as dairy products, whole wheat, and corn are regular culprits. In case your alleviation changes, then continue your brand-new diet. They could also provide several food sensitivities.

If you're breastfeeding, you may even need to temporarily remove these food types from your daily diet as well. Baby can still get smaller amounts of the food contaminants through your dairy.

6. Acid Reflux

While every baby encounters some spit up, babies who have forcefully shown spitting up and distress when being deposit may be experiencing acid reflux.

If your child is arching their back, squirming uncomfortably, and screaming when deposit, then this uncomfortable problem may be the culprit. This might also be the situation if they're not giving an answer to regular comfort or calmed with a swaddle.

You might be in a position to relieve this pain by lessening the quantity of dairy your child gets at each feeding. If you're breastfeeding, you'll be making too much dairy, and if your child is overeating, their stomachs are struggling to take all that dairy. You can even help lessen this by keeping your child upright for thirty minutes after eating. But also, inform your paediatrician if you believe your child has acid reflux disorder or allergies.

7. Transitioning Through Rest Cycles

Your body naturally undergoes phases of deep and light

sleep. There are occasions during the night where you will be awakened for just mere seconds before dosing off to rest, perhaps without memory from it.

That is natural and related to REM sleep and circadian rhythms. A baby must learn ways to get themselves back again to rest after these brief stages of waking and thinking. Your child might awake and crave the rocking, or relax prop, they've become familiar with when drifting off to sleep, and this is why your child doesn't't seem to remain asleep for a long length of time.

An excellent cure for this is to let your child layout when they may be sleepy, but awake to get accustomed to the sensation of drifting off for the reason of the environment, the mind then begins to create rest organizations and cues.

8. Baby is Hungry for Solid Food

Depending on how old they are, if they're over six months, their digestive tract may be craving more food. Milk provides proper nourishment, but their stomachs may need something more to utilize. Try presenting more solid food to their diet little by little and find out if indeed they stay full for much longer; if your child doesn't drink or eat as much any longer, please read our article about this.

9. It's Too Hot or Too Chilly for Baby

If your child is getting up during the night or oversleeping, check their bodies for sweat and hands for cold fingertips. This is a simple solution with their evening waking. Infants need just a little extra comfort than us to be comfortable and could want an extra blanket. Ideally, an infant is preferred in an area heat range of 68-72 levels degree Fahrenheit.

10. Development of Spurts

You might have experienced growing pains when you were a kid or teen, and babies have them too. Baby might proceed through per week of having a more enormous appetite to support this growth. They could also be awakened in the centre of the night time hungrier.

An ever-growing baby may become sleepier, but

additionally, it may cause sleeplessness too. They might be more interested in playing when they're getting into a new developmental phase, which makes it harder to relax and fall asleep.

Around eight weeks is a typical time for infants to encounter what is called rest regression, where they'll wake up more often during the night, even if indeed they previously were sleeping fine.

If your child is still having difficulty sleeping, then don't give up your search for the answer. A lot of things can cause evening waking and trouble to settle babies, plus they require you to discover it on their behalf. Losing from sleep isn't healthy for your baby, so don't quit.

CHAPTER 2

Is Past Due Bedtimes Bad?

As children grow, they spend the majority of their time sleeping. Children under the age of two tend to rest over twelve hours each day, though this time range would reduce over time as they grow, their rest health will stay important throughout their lives. With that said, many parents question are *could there be a right or wrong time for kids to visit bed?'*

Your Child's Sleep Schedule

As you make an effort to find out the best sleeping plan for your son or daughter, you might find that going to sleep later to them is precisely what produces results. Even though many parents suppose that children with past due nights aren't getting the correct amount of rest, this isn't always true.

Though many sleep specialists don't encourage that parents should allow their children to sleep late frequently, many factors, however, determine if sleeping late is bad per individual baby

The primary goal for just about any parent and sleep specialist is to ensure that children are receiving a full night's rest overall, whatever time each goes to sleep.

Infants with Late Bedtimes

Parents with newborns undoubtedly know the struggle of looking to get into the groove of finding a workable rest plan for themselves and their baby. Often, parents could find themselves placing a baby to bed much later than expected.

Predicated on the widely kept notion that children need to rest at a particular time, these new parents often get concerned that babies with past due bedtimes aren't getting the rest they want while this might not be true if a baby isn't sleeping with respect to the suggested amount of time, that is, about 14 hours per day, past due bedtimes are flawlessly elegant if your child is well-rested.

Additionally, it is essential that parents of babies with past due bedtimes have to ensure that they help them stick to a regular wake/nap/bed routine. This stability is vital for infants as they develop.

Children with Past Due Bedtimes

The parent and the baby become accustomed to the rest schedule of the baby in the process of fixing a regular rest schedule as time goes by While a well-balanced plan is necessary for infants with past due bedtimes, additionally, parents need to comprehend when to upgrade this sleeping regularly.

Although the same truth to getting enough sleep and possessing a constant sleep schedule to connect with children with past due bedtimes, as your son or daughter grows older, they'll likely have to change to something new. With the beginning of daycare or college, you''ll need to begin waking your son or daughter up at a certain time, and that may translate into a youthful bedtime.

Getting Your Child to Bed at an earlier Time

Parents of children with late bedtimes often dread the day they would need to change their child's routine. Although it certainly won't happen in a single night with the right methods, parents can get their children on the right track to sleeping.

Use the pursuing tips to change your child's rest schedule:

Concentrate on their wake time: Children tend to get to sleep every time they want. Children with past due bedtimes are especially vulnerable to wanting to fall asleep later, as their inner clock has already been designed this way. Establish your places on waking your son or daughter up previously to help fight this wish to drift off later. Parents can begin resetting their child's internal clock a couple of weeks before college begins to ensure they may be well-rested and ready for their new routine.

Shift by thirty minutes almost every other day: The rest clock requires progressive change; kick starts this modification period by establishing their wake-up time thirty minutes earlier virtually every other day or every day. That is enough speed that allows them to drift off sooner.

Understand how much rest is needed. Depending on their age, your son or daughter may need pretty much rest. Research your facts and seek advice from a health care provider or rest specialist to ensure your child gets the right amount.

Set the build for rest: Spend both hours before bedtime, placing the build for sleep. This implies no consumer electronics, exercise, caffeine, and other things that may keep your son or daughter awake. Likewise, keeping their bedroom dark during this period will allow these to drift off faster.

How to Decipher if Your Son or Daughter isn't Sleeping enough

Parents of infants with late bedtimes often question how their children's sleeping behaviours are damaged as they grow. In some instances, children might not be getting enough rest, irrespective of when their bedtime is.

Are you worried your son or daughter 't sleeping enough? Look out for these signals:

Constantly rubbing the eyes or yawning: As infants spend the majority of their day sleeping, they are informing tale signs that they have to get more rest ASAP.

Constant irritability and crankiness: Most of us get just a little irritable if we haven't been sleeping well. The same holds for your son or daughter, however how old they might be.

Drifting off to sleep on brief car rides: If you notice that your son or daughter always knocks from a short trip in the automobile or stroller, they likely have to get more rest.

Acting sleepy after waking: Even if your son or daughter is awake, this does not imply that they had a restful rest. In some instances, they do not get enough rest; in others, the grade of rest is not adequate.

If you discover that your child is sleeping well, a past due bedtime is not a bad thing. So long as you are ensuring your son or daughter is well-rested and sticking with a routine, you as well as your baby are doing just fine.

Chapter 3

Concerned about Baby's First Daycare Trip? 10 Ideas to Ease the Stress

For every mother or father who is going to leave their baby in a daycare for the very first time:

Are you taking your child to daycare for the very first time? One thousand questions must be running right through your brain. You are going to leave the infant you created inside you under the treatment of daycare educators. *Are you frightened?* That's normal because this milestone you are going to mix is no laughing matter.

The first couple of days would be the most difficult because both you and the tiny one will be transitioning into uncharted territory. As time passes, things are sure to get better, and you'll realize that this is the most sensible thing for both of you. Besides, sooner or later, you''ll have to slice the cord, right?

It's hard to show how this will continue to work away,

but with just a little preparation, going for the baby to daycare will be smoother than you imagined. Here's how to get ready for your baby's first-time at daycare.

Suggestions for the Parent

Every mother or father has read a horror tale regarding how an infant was staying in daycare, and things went south. Leaving your child in the treatment of a "stranger" is a problematic reality that each mother, dad, or guardian encounters sooner or later.

If you're thinking about taking your child to daycare, these pointers will ease the knowledge.

1. Do your homework

Nothing at all beats preparation than comprehensive research. Ask the daycare company as many questions as possible. If you spend sufficient time looking to discover the best service, you'll be at tranquillity, knowing that your son or daughter is under care. Do not shy away from trusting that gut feeling you have as soon as you head into the daycare.

What factors do you consider whenever choosing a

daycare?

✓ *Low caregiver-child ratio.*

✓ *Location: maybe it's near to work or home.*

✓ *The opening and closing times.*

✓ *Whether meals are included or not.*

✓ *Every other priority you might have.*

2. Create a checklist a night before daycare time

Many daycare veterans will let you know that one of the essential things to enhance your baby's stay in daycare is remembering to pack every item the baby might need. Infants need crib bedsheets, pacifiers, labelled containers, bibs, and other activities. Make a daycare checklist and stick it close to the door or behind your mobile phone.

3. Be positive at the drop-off

Children quickly grab their parent's disposition. If you're depressed and sulky throughout your baby's first-time at daycare, she or he will see it. Be intentional with your disposition, and be sure you project optimism.

4. Do some regular check-ins

Allowing someone else to provide for your child might cause you to feel just like you lost your control. It is even hard to start your daily responsibilities because you retain wondering the way they are faring. After taking your child to daycare, do some regular check-ins before pick-up time. It'll offer you a glance at how your baby gets along. Also, develop a good rapport with the educators.

5. Make the pick-up exciting

When collecting your son or daughter after taking your child to daycare, focus on linking with her or him at night. Provide them with a warm hug and a broad smile. Your baby will feel liked and will recognize that being in daycare is not a bad thing.

Tips For Your Child

Regardless of how old they are, babies likewise have a hard time transitioning into daycare. Fortunately, there are ways to help ease the tension on their behalf, such as these pointers.

1. Take the kid for a meet-and-greet

Before taking your child to daycare for the very first time, organized to allow them to meet their teachers beforehand. Spending time alone with someone not used to being family in your existence will help them to familiarise themselves with their surroundings. It will ease the changeover.

2. Provide them with a familiar object

Just a little feel of your house can make a baby's first time at a daycare easy to bear. Whatever smells or feels as though the home is all they might need to have them through their first day. Maybe it's a blanket, a toy, or a laminated face.

3. Explain what's happening

Even if your child hasn't started speaking yet, you can

still speak to her or him about the daycare. Discuss other kind aunties' care for them. Be sure you talk about the new playmates because they'll love that!

4. Get your child to rest early

The night time before taking your child to daycare establish how well they adapt to the new phase of their lives. Having sufficient sleep means that the kid is well-rested and can deal with the challenges that might confront the baby. An exhausted child is only going to make things harder than they are already. Ensure that the infant sleeps early almost every other night.

5. Introduce the idea gradually

After your baby's first-time at daycare goes well, you may be excited and want to take them the next time. However, this isn't a highly recommended move to make. For the first few times of taking the infant to daycare, take the kid on another basis. Introducing a fresh concept slowly allows sufficient time for your baby to get accustomed to the environment. It will reduce resistance.

Bonus suggestion: Tears are okay

Your baby's first-time at daycare may not be all flossy and smooth. It could take time for a kid to adjust to daycare. During this period, expect some tears from both the child and yourself. Sometimes the feelings might heighten during fall off while in other situations, it could be during the grab. Everyone must decompress when the problem is seemingly overpowering, as well as your baby may not know every other way besides crying. Those tears also tag a substantial milestone for your baby, which explains why you must embrace them.

They could adapt much better than you imagined

A baby's first-time at daycare doesn't have to be complicated. There's a high likelihood that your child will adjust much better than you think. As time passes, the sadness you feel will subside, and you'll be happy to have made a decision. Taking your child to daycare is an excellent learning experience.

Chapter 4

Ideas to Set up a Bedtime Regimen for Your Baby

A pleasurable bedtime routine assists children in easing the changeover from being awake to drifting off to sleep. An excellent regular bedtime can help your son or daughter feel convenient and secure in what to anticipate when each day concludes. To be able to build a regular bedtime for babies, you will need to build up a predictable series of activities that can undoubtedly and regularly be honoured each night.

The bedtime routine involved can begin to evolve and change as the kid starts to grow, although its basics should remain as these were right from the start. Based on your child's age group, the infant bedtime regular may involve putting on their PJs, cleaning their tooth, and then reading them a fascinating bedtime story.

Alternatively, the kid bedtime routine could also involve going for a bath, singing, or hearing a song, accompanied by another song, and a warm glass of water. As a mother or father, it is when you to produce a decision about how to make a bedtime regular. You also decide on if the night regular will stop wasting time and comfortable, or whether it will require a longer time that will help your relationship with your son or daughter.

A bedtime program idea will typically work best when you have reserved at least one hour before bedtime for participating in peaceful play with your son or daughter. Booking this timeframe helps lower the baby's activity levels while also planning their anxious system for a few much-needed relaxations.

Watching action-packed TV shows, taking part in tickling games, operating, and even roughhousing can make a peaceful changeover to sleep very hard for a child. If you're searching for a reasonable bedtime regular for children, consider the next illustrations. You can choose any bedtime regular that you think will continue to work best for your son or daughter:

Set a particular Time-table and be Sure to Stay with it

A child's body can modify a lot more easily to the bedtime regular if you select a bedtime regular that follows a constant and natural design. This means that you should avoid making changes to the night consistent as it'll make it even harder for the kid to drift off.

Give a Warning

Just before the kid must rest, be sure to issue a caution to the point that your day has begun to wind down. Based on your child's age group, they might be too young to start judging time at this time, which means that informing them five minutes to visit may as well not always do the job. However, you can instruct your child through association.

This is attained by starting the first area of the baby bedtime routine, e.g., putting the playthings away or using the bathing water. Choose how you desire to begin the bedtime regular, to be able to do the transmission that your day has started to wind down.

You can find parents who often choose to signal impending bedtime routine by getting the kitchen timer ring for 5 minutes; for a kid, this can be an indication that their bedtime is here. It also permits an opportunity in which a third party announces bedtime, therefore reducing the desire to have a kid to complain. It is because small children also recognize that it isn't possible to claim with machines.

Offer Your Son or Daughter a Snack

Light snacks, including carbohydrates and protein, for instance, half of the whole wheat or whole loaf of bread and a little bit of cheese, can help induce rest in a child and will allow the child to remain asleep for all of those other nights.

This is a perfect child bedtime routine, as the carbohydrates can help make the infant sleepy, while proteins, on the other hand, will ensure that your child's blood sugar reaches or remains level until breakfast time. Also, ensure that your baby cleans his/her tooth after eating.

Give Your Child a Warm Bath

It's important to make a bedtime program that also includes a warm shower. By increasing the child's body's temperature, you make the kid more susceptible to drifting off to sleep. Also, obtaining a chance to try out with her shower playthings will also get her to relax.

Getting Dressed for Bed

Another regular bedtime idea involves getting the child ready for bed. Because of this, you'll need to dress the infant using comfortable but nonbinding PJs. Make sure that the pyjamas are neither too light nor too warm.

Read a Tale to Your Child

That is one of the very most comforting and rewarding

bedtime routines for children. That is way more if the story plot in question is undoubtedly a favourite tale commonly associated with going to sleep, e.g., Goodnight Moon. However, take note that as the kid starts to develop, they'll want usage of more stories and also to a wider variety.

Play Soft Music

You can always incorporate soft music into the bedtime routine for babies. With gentle music, there is no need to do much as whatever you should do is to allow music play in the backdrop, watching as your son or daughter begins to drift off to slumberland.

Provide Your Son or Daughter with a Sleeping Buddy

When developing your child bedtime routine, you can test to include snuggle buddies into that routine. Here, a teddy bear or favourite doll comes into useful play in providing the comfort that your child needs.

Eliminate or Limit Bottles

If your child has previously needed a container to be able to drift off, ensure that in the new child bedtime schedule, the bottle is only going to contain water. Juice method or dairy will usually pool around his tooth leading to the introduction of cavities, which may be dangerous, specifically for small children.

Make Sure Your Goodnights are Brief

You need to make a bedtime schedule that will truly see you only say goodnight when it's time for both parents to leave the child's room. While at it, try very difficult not to return even if the kid calls out for you. This might sound severe, but each time you get back to the area when the kid calls you, you begin conditioning your son or daughter to discover that parents will usually keep coming back quickly when they may be called.

For just about any bedtime schedule, the proven fact is that you appear strict to ensure that it's followed to the notice. Any hesitation on your end can be found by the kid to imply that you weren't seriously interested in her going to sleep. it shows them that if indeed they yell out for you truly loudly, you should have no option but to return and check out them.

Be Patient

As with some other new activity, it's essential to exercise some persistence. For your brand-new baby bedtime program, you might have to arrange for it at least fourteen days in advance. Recognise that it will require some time for this to take hold essentially. When you are exercising this new bedtime regularly, you'll need to ensure that all persons who are usually to be involved in placing the infant to bed are just about every night and working towards making sure the new system takes hold.

Have a Chat

Bedtime is always a good time that you can spend a few moments talking to your child. It isn't mandatory that you wait before the baby is old enough to begin narrating the occasions that occurred throughout the day. You can sit by his/her crib and relate how your entire day went. That is a terrific way to get your child to relax and drift off without leading to a fuss.

Make Sleep a Family Priority

You can perform this by identifying how much sleep is necessary for each person. Once determined, ensure that they all have enough rest. If there are any problems, ensure that they are talked about with your small children's doctor. Many such issues are often treated.

Stick to Your Child Bedtime Routine

If the toddler tries to e their boundaries, you'll need to be kind but the company as well. Being a parent, it'll be essential to ensure that you adhere to what you have said. If not, your child could keep pressing the limitations until you finally quit.

Which means that you might have to repeat the procedure as many times as necessary. Furthermore, try to resist the desire to show discomfort or get upset with the toddler's attempts to lengthen their bedtime. Getting angry or showing discomfort only means that the whole process is sure to get prolonged.

The Takeaway

Just like there are numerous methods for getting your child to drift off, there are specific things that you can avoid, if not your son or daughter will end-up developing poor sleeping habits. It's important to note that whenever there is nothing done, many infants who have developed poor sleeping practices when young will continue steadily to have the same issues when they start going to school. You will need to handle your child's sleeping practices from an early age. Please remember, if your son or daughter is not getting enough rest, then neither are you.

Chapter 5

Will Controlled Crying Work? Benefits and Drawbacks

When you just give birth to a baby, sleep becomes an extravagance, especially for the first couple of weeks. If you don't have help and are managing the complete change on your own, you will probably find yourself sleepwalking.

The majority of parents do some searching online for tips to get the infant to sleep. Sleep is essential for the infant, and performing lullabies might not always assist with the sleeplessness situation. That is why we have physicians and organizations promoting rest/sleep training as a means of helping infants get themselves to rest/sleep earlier.

With this process, your toddler would not only go to sleep with reduced hitches but also the wakes in the centre of the night time will be minimal.

A couple of two sleep training methods: "controlled crying" and "cry it away" approach. Before adopting either technique, you should seek advice from your pediatrician to determine which is right for the infant.

Before considering the training methods, it's essential to ensure that the infant is of good health, well-fed, and is not looking for a diaper change. In this chapter; we are discussing managed crying and exactly how it helps infants get themselves to rest.

What is Controlled Crying?

Controlled crying is a favourite rest/sleep training approach suggested by Richard Ferber back the 1980s. This technique aims at assisting a kid get him/herself to rest without developing any long-term results that could affect his/her health.

When working with this, your child will drift off without you singing a lullaby or soothing him/her. This technique looks to make your son or daughter liable for his/her sleeping habits.

Even if you get hurt hearing the infant cry, you have to apply some tough love for better sleep habits. If done correctly, you might fix your child's test schedule. However, the effectiveness depends on this and the health of the kid.

Newborns tend to be awake often at night time for a diaper change and feeding. So, if you would like to try this out, the infant needs to be at least six months old. Furthermore, you have to ensure that the infant is within good health since a fever or other problems could cause restlessness and continuous crying, thus reducing the potency of the whole process. Make sure to give food to the infant well and change a moist diaper to ensure maximum comfort while attempting this approach.

How It's Done

The theory is to help an infant sleep by him/herself

without your comfort. For this to work, the managed crying is often followed by managed comforting as a means of looking into and reassuring the kid. In some instances, if the child persists the cry, you might stroke his/her mind or sing a lullaby to make calmness. Yet, you should leave the area while the young child continues to be awake for the training to reach your goals.

Step 1: Leave.

The first rung on the ladder into practicing this process is to leave the infant awake in the cot. Say goodnight to him/her and then gradually exit the area.

When you leave, expect the toddler to cry a lot since he/she is not used to the abandonment.

Step 2: Wait.

If the infant is constantly on the cry, wait at least two minutes prior to going back inside. Once there, reassure the kid that everything is alright before exiting the area after only a few minutes.

Step 3: Check.

If more than five minutes elapse and the infant continues to cry, return inside for the intended purpose of reassurance. When you say goodnight and leave the area for another time, supply the baby seven to eight minutes before going inside if he/she continues to cry. Keep duplicating this process and present a period of two more minutes every time you leave the area prior to going inside.

The much longer you leave the infant in this new process, the greater he/she will figure out how to sleep without your presence.

Is Controlled Crying Safe for my Baby?

Yes, it is safe for infants because they learn how to place themselves to settle in your absence. As time passes, they will overcome the shock to be abandoned, and the thought of sleeping independently is strengthened in their thoughts.

However, before you begin, you should ensure that the toddler is full, not thirsty, not ill, and the diaper is transformed. You have to know whether your child has extreme parting anxiousness, which happens once you leave him/her only. If he/she does, then it is incomparably a tough time because the best training might be considered a little harder.

The drawback of the method is that you'll have to abandon your kid and make her or him to cry without you comforting her or him. Some individuals believe that this may cause infants problems in the foreseeable future. However, none of this has shown that.

There is follow-up research conducted in 2012 by the Official Journal of the American Academy Of Paediatrics on the impact of the particular sleep training method; the analysis showed that it is a safe rest training technique without long-lasting aftereffect for the babies.

Moreover, managed crying comes strongly suggested by NHS as a means of supporting address short-to-medium-term issues like major maternal depression and sleep issues in infants.

How to Manage Controlled Crying

For some parents, managed crying could make them emotional because they need to pay attention to the kid as he or she cries. You will likely cave in, following the first trial; that is why we advise that you seek support from your lover or a trusted friend. In this manner, every time you feel like picking right up the young child through the training period, you can call somebody who will restrain you.

Your friend or partner will also help if you are getting a bad day as the baby's crying reaches you. If you relapse, your time and efforts will be inadequate.

There is absolutely no point in trying this on the toddler today and skipping the schedule tomorrow. For efficiency, you will need to get a new continuous program. Therefore the child gets used to the changes.

You'll achieve greater results when the infant is sleepy and just a little tired. Furthermore, ensure that the kid is not in problems before or in this rest training process.

How Long would Controlled Crying Last?

Different infants respond differently to various treatments. That is also the situation with managed crying. A couple of babies who have no issue sleeping, as well as for them, this process will almost certainly last between four to five times. When this happens, you are only going to have to tolerate hearing your child cry for a brief period to be able to help him or her rest better by himself or herself.

However, some infants experience sleeping problems in a

way that you'll need to tolerate the crying for approximately two weeks for this to begin working.

If this era is over, as well as your baby still cries much without sleeping, then it could be time that you vary from manipulated crying to some other approaches. You can seek advice from your pediatrician who'll help identify the best option sleep training way for your baby.

The Benefits

One of the primary benefits of practicing this in infants is to instill a new skill in them. This means that the young child will understand how to visit sleep by him/herself without help. That is helpful to both child and mother or father.

Another benefit is that it's instant and effective in infants with healthy sleeping habits. Some infants learn to rest independently after only two evenings of managed crying, while some may take just a little longer.

Parents and guardians who've successfully been able to rest train their infants using the managed crying technique declare that the method works well. It will help to lessen settling, as well as waking problems experienced by infants. Infants who've undergone this technique tend to rest far better on a short-term basis compared to the other infants.

The Drawbacks

Managed crying has some disadvantages, and one of these is creating stress on the mother or father.

You may feel guilty:

It is tough to relax and pay attention to the child cry without picking him/her up. You, therefore, have to be continual and courageous if you would like to sleep and teach your baby effectively. This, however, might be considered a problem for a few parents because they don't want to live with the guilt of allowing the infant to cry.

The infant may disturb others:

If you live with other families, a crying child may cause disruption, thus causing this to be method unsuitable for you because of the emotions of abandonment that the kid might develop after crying only, some experts claim that managed crying could cause some psychological problems later in life. Nevertheless, it has not shown.

It could make your child sick:

The other drawback is that some babies might become ill after too much crying.

Chapter 6

7 Ways to Turn-over Your Child from a Crib to a Toddler Bed

You'll inevitably have to changeover your son or daughter from a crib to a bed sooner or later! They can't set off to university still sleeping in their crib! But, when and how can you make the changeover? You want your child to figure out how to rest in their bed but tend to know when to make the big move from a crib to a bed. Additionally, you want to ensure that the changeover from a crib to a kid's bed is as painless as easy for both you, as well as your child. Below, we have some information to help you select when, as well as how to help move your son or daughter from a crib to a bed.

Signs Your Son or Daughter is Preparing to Proceed to a Young Child's Bed

It might be time to help make the changeover from a crib to a bed under the following circumstances:

Climbing: If your son or daughter has begun climbing away from their crib, it could be time to take them off their crib to a kid's bed. However, if your son or daughter has only climbed from the crib one time, it might not be time to help make a move at this time. Some kids climb out once and then don't climb out again for a long time.

Your son or daughter is requesting a huge kid's bed: If your son or daughter has begun to verbalize for you that they need their own big kid's bed, it could imply that they will be ready to make a move.

You will be ready to night potty-train: If you're along the way of potty-training and believe that your kid is preparing to make it during the night without having a major accident, you might move your kid to a toddler bed to allow them to access the toilet.

You have another baby along the way soon:

Sometimes, the reason why you thought you would move your son or daughter from a crib to a bed may be more significantly regarding you than your son or daughter. When you have another baby along the way and will need the crib for your brand-new baby soon, it could be time to move your child to the bed. You'll want to get this to move sometime before you have the newborn, which means that your toddler doesn't have to adapt to both a fresh bed and a fresh sibling at the same time.

How to Ensure a Steady Transition to the Brand New Bed

Once you've determined that it's time to change over your son or daughter from a crib to a bed, there are several things you should think about before you plunge in and make the big move.

Stay away from arranging the move when other big changes or transitions are happening:

If there are other big changes occurring in your toddler's life, you will likely want to carry off on moving them from a crib to a bed for some time. If your child has just begun daycare or preschool, you're starting to potty-train, or you're planning for a trip someplace that will interrupt your schedule, it could be a much better idea to hold back a while to help make the transition.

The keeping of the brand new Bed

Your child is used to the positioning where they sleep each evening; they are accustomed to getting the same view of the lover in their room, the curtains, and their nightlight, make an effort to keep this as similar as you possibly can by putting their bed in the same location as their crib. This can help make the move from a crib to a bed easier on your child (and you).

Purchase special books to learn together

There are numerous books that have been written that can help to make the transition from a crib to a bed easier on your baby. These books help simplify your child's worries and have them excited to settle their big childbed. Some titles you can consider are "A Bed of your," "Big Enough for a Bed," and "I enjoy Sleep in my Bed."

Involve your son or daughter in selecting their new bed and bedding

Help get your child excited and committed to having a fresh, big kid's bed. Make sure they are an integral part of the procedure of selecting and establishing their new bed. Bring them shopping with you when you intend to choose the new bed. If you wish to make the options just a little less mind-boggling to them, you can offer them several options to choose from (this may also help make sure that you are alright with the bed they choose).

You can even let them choose new bedding for the new big kid's bed. Maybe, choose a few new, coordinating adornments for his or her bedroom too. They'll be more motivated to settle their bed if indeed they feel like that they had a job in creating it!

Re-evaluate your childproofing

Before you make the big move from a crib to a toddler bed, you should re-examine their room. You'd likely have to childproofed the area, but that should be before the kids are heading to being capable of getting out of their bed in the center of the night time without you being there. Check that there aren't any potential hazards in the area. Ensure that all their furniture are installed to the wall structure. Consider placing a gate in their doorway, so they don't get access to all of those other rooms in the center of the night time. Do all you can to ensure they'll be safe in their room if indeed they let themselves out of bed.

Stick to your present bedtime routines

To make sure you have a smooth changeover for your son or daughter, it will be very important to stick to your present bedtime routines. You'll have to keep everything as regular as possible to help your son or daughter adapt to their new bed. If you don't now have a constant bedtime, it may be beneficial to create one before you make an effort to move your son or daughter from a crib to a bed.

Be patient and provide comfort

Moving from a crib to a young child bed is a huge change for your little man or gal. Show patience and comfort them if they're scared or anxious. You can test sharing some occasions when you've been worried and what you do to do yourself a favour to complete the tough times.

Moving your child from a crib to a bed can be a huge adjustment for you both. With some uniformity and planning, though, your child will prepare yourself and be excited to help make the big change.

Chapter 7

Why do some Infants Cry During Sleep?

You've probably experienced this situation often as a fresh parent. Your child has been asleep for one hour, maybe two, when abruptly she cried out in her rest. Understandably, you might feel puzzled or worried about why your child is crying while asleep.

However, most times, there is absolutely no reason behind alarm if an infant cries during sleep. Many reasons can mae a child cry while asleep. Here's the scoop on why your child begins to cry.

Sleep Cycles

Relating to working Mom, your child has rest cycles that run for approximately 50 to 60 minutes per routine, (unlike you who undergoes your rest cycles about every 90 minutes roughly).

Each cycle has a transitional phase, where the sleeper - in cases like this, your child - techniques in one phase to some other. Of these transitions, say whenever your baby techniques from REM to a more profound rest routine, he/she may cry out.

Whenever a baby cries during sleep, it is a sign that his/ her rest cycles are transitioning. In every actuality, your child isn't awake. Like just about everything else, an infant must understand how to do, he/ she must understand how to drift off properly and also stay asleep.

Other Challenges

Granted, while most of the time, an infant cries during sleep because of rest change, you know well that he/ she may be experiencing other issues. Your child could be, for example, starving or damp.

So, how will you know why your child is crying while asleep? Healthline offers this little bit of advice when you're thinking about "How come my baby is crying during sleep?"

If, after a few moments, your baby's cries escalate rather than calming down, you should understand that there is surely an issue.Simply know that if your child is transitioning in one rest cycle to some other, his/ her cries won't escalate.

However, if your child cries during sleep and he/ she seems increasingly more distressed, it's time for you to go check up on your child. As we've already mentioned, the infant could be damp or starving or even chilly, and undoubtedly, sick.

Problems to Sleep

Without knowing it, you can inadvertently cause your child to be awakened at night time. A baby is named a "trained night time crier," based on the Children's Medical center Colorado.

Your child should create a regular seven or eight-hour sleeping routine by the ages of eight weeks to four months. By this time, your baby's caloric needs change: he/she will no more require calories at night time and, thus, won't need nocturnal feedings.

If you're questioning why your child cries during sleep after about age four weeks, you will see that we now have some very common triggers because of this.

You should entertain your child after he/she wakes up. Preferably, you should help your child get accustomed to a more resolved regular bedtime. After tale time has ended and the infant has dropped asleep, don't get the books back out again or play with your child. Even constant rocking at nap time can teach your child to be awaken while asleep and weep. Crying while asleep if it happens on the standard could be a sign that your child has a second gain from getting up. In other words, he/ she needs to be interested or is planning to be dependent on mother and dad's attention.

You rock your child to make him/ her drift off. Granted, in the initial phases of life, an infant must be rocked and soothed to be able to drift off. However, one of your targets as a mother or father ought to be to educate your child on how to self-regulate. An excellent sleeper in the infant years may become a good sleeper in old age. If your child cries during sleep, maybe it's a sign that he/ she doesn't learn how to drift off without rocking.

Your baby gets used to changes in the environment or routine. Babies cannot chat the way people can; unlike you, your child must cry to connect. The crying that originates from these changes is named "protest crying." It's the natural consequence of a significant change that your child doesn't like.

Must I call the Physician if my Baby can't Sleep?

The easy, most maddening response to this is, "This will depend."

If the crying is relatively recent and doesn't appear to be escalating, it's probably just normal nighttime rest transition crying. If it's escalating and you've attempted feeding your child or changing him/her diaper or whatever, then you might have a far more serious issue.

Sometimes, your child can form reflux. If he/she spits up quite a little or is wheezing, you might want a checkup.

That said, additionally, it is okay to get active support from your physician as you find out about your child. If your child cries during sleep, it could be nothing. It might also be considered an indication of something much more serious. If you'is prone to getting worried,go on and give yourself the satisfaction that will come from a call to your baby's doctor.

In conclusion; if your child cries during sleep, maybe it's an indicator of something serious. However, it might also just imply that he/she is transitioning from one stage of the rest cycle to some other. (Your child has rest cycles as everyone else does). Frequently, trying to look for the reason behind crying while asleep is why most parents get frustrated.

Usually, your child will cry away at night time for brief intervals, often due to a change in the sleep cycle, but also as a consequence of hunger, wetness, or cold. The best way to determine the difference between these numerous kinds of cries is to pay attention to escalation. If your child cries during sleep but stops after a few moment and the crying doesn't get more immediate, it's probably a rest cycle thing.

However, if the crying gets louder or even more insistent, then it's time to check on for other issues. Many parents that face this matter find themselves being surprised to discover that their infants have never woken up, regardless of the crying.

Too much fussing over the infant for night-crying can result in a baby to become night crier. In cases like this, an infant cries during sleep because your child has a second gain from getting up. Quite only, if your child has found that he/she will reach play or get a mother or dad's attention, keeping asleep will end up being difficult.

Finally, some sleep issues arise from medical ailments like reflux. Having your physician check your child out will get rid of the worry it causes you whenever your baby cries during sleep.

Remember, letting your child cry for a few moments after he/she has fallen asleep isn't precisely like making him/her cry throughout the day. Often, these daytime cries reveal something much more severe or are your baby's way of interacting with you. Understanding how to distinguish between the types of cries that your child produces will eventually help everyone get some good, much-needed sleep.

Chapter 8

8 Methods to manage the Sleep Schedule of Two Children

As a fresh parent of the baby, it has already been challenging enough to get your baby to sleep. Now imagine wanting to dual this challenge with the addition of another child. If you're a mother or father of twins or your kids are sleeping collectively, it might appear impossible to change both children's sleep schedules to work harmoniously. Fortunately, where there's a will, there's a way. This is the connection with parents who have been successful in handling their two kid's rest schedules.

Get help! Handling two kid's sleep schedules can be considered a challenge for an individual parent or a few. The first weeks of the life span of your infants will require all your time merely to manage their sleeping routines.

Ensure you get help in early stages, and acknowledge offers from relatives and friends for assistance with chores around the house and operating errands. In this manner, you'll be exclusively concentrated on caring for your children.

Putting kids to Sleep Simultaneously

Even if your kids are sleeping on different mattresses, you can put them right down to rest at exactly the same time. Achieving this will ensure that both of them have the same sleeping tempo that their body will eventually tune into.

Feed Both at the same time

Exactly like with putting children to rest jointly, feeding them jointly will teach their bodies to wake them up at some aspects of the night time specifically for meals. Even if one of the kids is not awake, give food to them immediately after you have given the first one. In this manner, your twins' rest schedules will synchronize, and they'll learn to be awaken for eating at exactly the same time.

Even though you do not feel it is to awaken a snoozing baby, it's the only means of avoiding jumping backward and forwards between two children at night time.

Separate Them

If one of the twins is old enough and seems prepared to sleep through the entire night without getting up to consume, you can temporarily move he/her to another room.

When you have to, accommodate one of your loveable space for the sleeping twin so the other will not wake up during the night. When the waking twin is preparing to forget about night meals, both can be cut back together in a single room.

Have a Regular Bedtime Routine

Developing a bedtime routine is essential when you

yourself have an infant. It becomes even more necessary whenever there are two. A bedtime regular can contain:

- ✓ Playing comforting games.

- ✓ Reading a bedtime story.

- ✓ Massage.

- ✓ Bath time.

- ✓ Dim lights.

- ✓ Soft music.

A routine is a way to let your kids know to affiliate certain events with bedtime. Maybe it's the water operating or the lighting heading dim that let them know that enough time to rest is soon. When these routines are repeated every day, they'll become ingrained into the children's rest habits. Their brain will naturally start to associate certain activities with sleeping. This gives a feeling of security and comfort to them besides assisting them rest during the night.

Two times Feeding Schedule

To synchronize your twins' rest schedules, it is essential

to give food to them at the same time as well. Infants who are given together will fall asleep collectively.

Utilizing a Lovey

When it is safe, you can start adding a lovey into the children's cribs. Be sure you follow the rules for a safe lovey before placing anything next to your children's sleeping surface. Find a little and safe lovey, which makes smooth sounds. This assists the infants to associate the mild feel and audio with rest time.

Start Early with Twins

While a single child does not require to indeed have a set routine until about five or six months, the situation with twins' rest routine requires that you begin early. Although arriving home from a healthcare facility may as well not be the most likely moment to commence with, consider starting a twins' rest schedule but as soon as four to six weeks. After per month, it'll already be apparent that you'll require to start out arranging your two children's rest schedules to be able to get rest for yourself as well as your children.

Some times things might not go according to plan, work to generate predictability into the two kid's rest schedules. This implies developing the twins' rest schedules in early stages so that it becomes ingrained into them by enough time when they are small children.

Follow Your Tempo

Much like any advice, you have to think about your unique situation. In case your two children's rest schedules do not frustrate you, there is no need to begin off so early. However, parents who are used to two kid's rest schedules advise controlling your twins' rest schedules as soon as possible. While controlling the rest of one child can be placed off, two children's rest schedules going in various directions really can take the life span out of you eventually.

In conclusion; feel the right path into the two kid's rest schedules, and consider if you are ready to mind down this street. Controlling your twins' rest schedules brings incredible rewards for you as a mother or father and also to both your kids. When their schedules will be the same, they'll no more wake one another up, and you'll have two happy children and parents to thank for it.

Chapter 9

8 Common Baby Sleep Myths

In that first couple of months of new parenthood, everything can appear, such as a blur of exhaustion. You might feel like you do everything incorrectly, and you're sure to get a lot of advice, both solicited and unsolicited.

One subject matter that it appears everyone comes with a judgment on is rest. Advice about rest is so popular and so mixed it can feel impossible to split up reality from baby rest myth. Improving rest is very important to both parents and the infant so that it is important to comprehend some common myths and separate misconceptions from fact.

Separating Baby Sleep Myth from Fact

Myth 1: *Infants need to be place down in a completely calm and dark room to sleep.*

Truth: Your child will quickly figure out how to rest in whatever environment he's subjected to. He might actually rest better when there is certainly activity happening around him, as it could create some sort of white noise.

Myth 2: *You shouldn't expect your child to sleep well for weeks or even the first year.*

Truth: Infants can figure out how to rest well in only a few weeks. Doing this takes work on your part, and it could be annoying but will lead to better rest for everybody. Teaching rest cues, or methods that your child learns to associate with rest, such as swaddling, is a superb way to boost rest patterns.

Myth 3: *Infants wake up at night time because they have to eat.*

Truth: Once your child is between four and six months old, if he's gaining weight, he's thriving physically, and if the mom is medical, there are no issues with dairy supply, you don't have for your child to awaken to eat.

Myth 4: *Medical or rocking can make it impossible to really get your baby to rest some other way.*

Truth: Your child will need what he/she is utilized to, that is natural. But there is certainly nothing incorrect with rocking or nursing your son or daughter to rest. They key is to help him/her figure out how to put him/herself back again to rest when he wakes up. Supporting them learn self-soothing techniques allow them to place themselves back again to sleep at night time.

There are a number of behaviors you can encourage that teach your child to self-soothe, including:

✓ Sucking or cuddling a toy or blanket

✓ Utilizing a pacifier

✓ Humming softly, you can coach this by humming

softly as you rock and roll him.

✓ Stroking his hands or cheeks. Again, you can model this behavior for him if you are rocking or nourishing him.

Myth 5: *Reducing on day time naps will improve nighttime sleeping.*

Truth: That is a common thought, but it doesn't work. An excessively exhausted baby will be fussy plus much more difficult to access sleep when compared to a well-rested baby. Instead, make naps important, and begin the bedtime regular a little sooner than you think is essential which means you aren't rushed getting the baby to rest.

Myth 6: *Infants can go with a flexible routine, depending on the actual parents wish to accomplish.*

Truth: Sure, you can tote your child around wherever

you decide to go. If you wish to enhance the quality of rest for everybody, your loved ones, you should dedicate ultimately to developing a constant nap and bedtime regular. This might mean being near to home when you establish steady rest habits, but it'll pay back with an infant that would go to rest easily and sleeps well.

Myth 7: *Making an infant "cry it out" is harmful*

Truth: Studies show that there surely is no damage done by making your child cry it out during the night. If he's fed, dry and clean, and has a safe, comfortable crib, allowing him cry it out won't cause any problems.

However, that will not mean it's the only way to help your son or daughter sleep during the night. There are a number of ways to encourage sleeping during the night, and everything can succeed. If you're not comfortable allowing your child cry it out, there is absolutely no reason to use that approach to sleep training.

Myth 8: *Infants rest better if you put in a little cereal with their nighttime container.*

Truth: As stated above, a wholesome, growing baby doesn't need to awaken to consume. Adding cereal to his container isn't just unnecessary, but it additionally doesn't really work and can create other problems.

It isn't recommended to begin solids before six months old, and at that time, it ought to be within meals. Adding calorie consumption from cereal in a nighttime container can result in excessive putting on weight.

In conclusion; as you can plainly see, there are a great number of myths surrounding infants sleep behaviors and patterns. For each baby sleep misconception, you hear, there is certainly another that contradicts it. Keep in mind, as a mother or father, you should do what works for your household. If someone offers advice that noises beneficial, you can simply contemplate it, but make the possibilities by yourself. When you have questions or concerns, speak to your pediatrician.

Chapter 10

Breastfeeding isn't Always Easy: Most Common Problems & Solutions

Congratulations mommy! You've given birth to a lovely, bouncing baby girl or youngster. If you're anything like the majority of moms-to-be, you would have spent the last previous nine months learning and researching all there is certainly to learn about bringing an infant into this world.

Although a lot of the info and advice you received would be helpful but nothing can truly prepare you for what things to expect once your brand-new baby is home with you. As well as the preliminary shock of experiencing a little individual to care for each second of your day, the rest deprivation and hormone imbalances can make the first couple of days, weeks or even a few months of motherhood quite challenging.

Getting Baby Home & What to Expect

As stated previously, the first couple of days or weeks with your child can be hugely overwhelming. Once home, you quickly learn that life with an infant is nothing beats the advertisements on television. It really is significant amounts of work, so that as much as it is satisfying it's also exhausting.

As long as you have the assistance of the nurses on staff or simply your midwife. From here on, you are exclusively in charge of just a little human being that requires you for what appears to be every second of your day. It is an enormous learning curve that moms, both new and veteran must conquer.

Aside from dealing with *postpartum major depression and sleep deprivation*, one of the very most difficult transitions into motherhood is most likely conquering the artwork of breastfeeding. Like a mom, breastfeeding is considered to be among the best actions you can take for yourself as well as your baby. However, one of the principal issues that a lot of women face with medical is when their baby isn't emptying their breasts.

The Anxiety and Challenges of Breastfeeding for the very first time

Am i carrying this out right? My baby isn't emptying my breasts?

For many moms, understanding how to breastfeed their baby for the very first time could be very intimidating. You're exhausted, your child is screaming and isn't draining your breasts. If the last mentioned details you, don't fret, you aren't alone.

Breastfeeding can be quite challenging, and because of the anxiousness of everything, many moms, unfortunately, do not see it through to the finish. Initially, nursing your child will harm depending on your own threshold for pain. However, regardless of the latter, it'll get better.

With endurance and consistency, you'll get through it. For some moms, the first fourteen days are actually the most challenging. However, studies also have shown that if it is possible to make at night first couple of weeks, you will probably achieve success in your breastfeeding trip.

What do I really do when breastfeeding doesn't appear to be working?

Don't be ashamed to ask questions

If you're having difficulty with getting acclimated to your breastfeeding trip, please never hesitate to ask questions. Secondly, don't be stressed, You aren't alone. There are various resources as well as various organizations that offer problems with respect to breastfeeding.

Generally, in most U. S clinics there are lactation consultants that work carefully with moms before and after their pregnancy. Before you leave a healthcare facility, make certain to alert the personnel if your child isn't emptying your breasts. Before your real milk supply will come in you should have colostrum. Colostrum is quick dense and sometimes your child would have trouble extracting it.

Additionally, there is the non-profit organization *'La Leche League'* which targets providing education, advocacy as well as training for everything breastfeeding related. Every one of the above are reliable resources that are in spot to help you whenever you can.

Ensure that there is absolutely no underlying medical issue

There are a variety of reasons that might be triggering problems with nursing as well as perhaps why your child isn't draining your breast. Lots of the conditions that most moms face can be easily remedied at home using various natural techniques. However, one major reason which may be leading to issues with your child draining your breasts is actually a mechanized problem called "tongue connect".

A tongue tie occurs when the thin strip of tissues that connects the tongue to the ground of the mouth area is too brief. This issue can make it difficult for infants to suckle effectively. Due to the last mentioned, your breast will not really be drained effectively during feedings that will get them to engorged as well as your nipples sore. If you do believe that your child is experiencing a tongue-tie, the treatment will require the assistance of a medical expert.

Common explanations why your child isn't emptying your breast

The primary issue that a lot of women face when nursing is when their baby is not draining their breasts. The last mentioned could possibly be the consequence of lots of issues.

Here are some of the most typical reasons why your child isn't emptying your breasts effectively.

"My Baby just won't latch": It is rather common for

babies to have trouble latching for the very first time. Most infants are very sleepy a lot of the time, so you'll frequently have to do some motivating to encourage them to eat. When medical it's better to use the "nasal area to nipple technique".

After getting the baby into an appropriate breastfeeding position, place baby's nose on the nipple. The smell of your dairy or colostrum will stimulate and really should cause your child opening her mouth area to consume. Another technique you could attempt is expressing a little amount of dairy on your nipple and then putting it on baby's lip area. This will also help excite your baby to awaken and eat, as well as motivating effective draining of your breasts.

"When my baby will latch it's painful": As stated previously, breastfeeding can be somewhat unpleasant, especially initially. Unfortunately, there is absolutely no method that will completely get rid of the discomfort. You can find, however, lotions and even nipple shields

that will help relatively with the pain.

"My baby falls asleep after just a few minutes of medical": A terrific way to help your child awaken and eat is by using the "pores and skin to pores and skin" technique. Most moms have heard about the latter sooner or later during their being pregnant or throughout their postpartum period. Pores and skin to pores and skin causes the body release a prolactin, which is the hormone that helps the body produce dairy. If your child isn't draining your breasts because they're too sleepy, try undressing them. It's better to remove everything except the diaper.

Whenever your baby can feel your skin layer and smell your dairy, it'll cause her to "main" or seek out your breasts. Once latched, don't allow your child to drift off. Even if your child is actually starving, sometimes their wish to rest is higher than their will to remain up and eat.

Quick Mommy Suggestion: Take into account that all babies eat differently. Some infants are fast eaters; they'll be done within five to ten minutes, while some may require from thirty minutes to a complete hour before they may be full. Preventing the nursing program short, may be why your child isn't emptying your breasts thoroughly.

Clogged ducts: A clogged duct will surely be at fault in why your child isn't emptying your breast. A clogged duct in your breasts occurs when the encompassing tissue becomes swollen or swollen. You may even feel small lumps on your breasts that feel sore when handled.

To take care of the latter, try utilizing a warm compress accompanied by gently massaging your chest. Following the compress and therapeutic massage, you can also make an effort to hands express. Do these steps again normally as necessary before blockage is released, as well as your baby is draining your breasts properly. If you're working with a clogged duct, please don't let the problem prolong. A connected or clogged duct left neglected can cause contamination.

Be patient with your body as well as your baby

Breastfeeding won't continually be easy, you might perfectly have a few hurdles to climb before you get the suspend of it. However, don't quit. When you are dealing with an infant who isn't emptying your breasts or simply you're coping with latching issues, don't be anxious, it's not the end of the world.

Don't forget that you will not be alone. A lot of women have trouble at first with draining their breasts effectively. Be tolerance with the body, nothing at all happens right away. However, with a while and perseverance, you'll be a breastfeeding pro very quickly.

Chapter 10

Top 8 iPhone Apps to Really Get Your Child to Sleep

Getting a baby to sleep can be considered a tough job for a fresh mother or father. Sometimes, even the most experienced parents face the task of getting their infants to nap. However, some applications can help your child to drift off. This is what a perfect iPhone application to help children sleep can do for you:

- ✓ Help the infant sleep when fatigued enough
- ✓ Calm the newborn
- ✓ Help the infant rest for longer
- ✓ Soothe the newborn
- ✓ Get the infant ready for sleep
- ✓ Relax the newborn.

But obtaining a good baby sleep application can be hard. You can find dozens of applications with different functionalities, which will make choosing an application difficult. This list will slim down the list and make it easy so that you can choose an iPhone application to help children sleep.

1. Eat Sleep

On Apple store, this application lets you keep an eye on your baby's sleeping patterns. You are able to understand how long the newborn sleeps, that allows you to recognize any issues or patterns as they occur. If your child has sleeping issues, this application is ideal for assisting you determine them.

They have a note-taking feature that enables you to take notes like disease or teething. The application is so simple that anyone may use it. You merely require getting into the sleep start time and stop time. Also, you can include the nourishing information to obtain additional prominent general information about the sleep of the infant.

2. Baby Shusher

The Baby Shusher application utilizes the ancient shushing method. The idea behind the application form is that shushing noises assist in halting infants from crying and therefore soothe kids to sleep. When you have been shushing all day every day, this iPhone app is great for providing you a breather. It is effective with fussy infants.

The application has an attribute for setting the time that you would like the shushing to occur. It could be established for ranging from a quarter-hour and eight hours. If your child only responds to your tone of voice, you can record a custom shush, as well as your baby won't inform the difference. Furthermore, there's a great function that listens to the infant, and changes shush quantity accordingly. The application costs $4, which makes it a credible iPhone application to help children sleep.

3. Sound Sleeper

This application is free on the Apple store and it is a

perfect iPhone application to help children sleep. It depends on the infant's need to get over the world's silence. They have plenty of varied noises that you can choose to assist your child sleeping. A number of the noises include soft rainfall sound, active market noises, and the audio of the car's operating engine. Based on your child, you can pick the sound you know they'll like.

White noise is popular for helping children to drift off, and the application comes with an option for replicating sounds that are usually inside the womb. They have three settings: Play, to assist the infant in drifting off to sleep; Pay attention for assisting the infant to stay asleep; Track to assist you in being current with your baby's sleeping patterns. Through the Pay attention mode, the application will know when the infant wakes up and begins to cry, and it'll immediately start calming the baby to stay to sleep.

Sound sleeper gives you to control the quantity of each audio. However , if you download the pay version, you'll be able to control the space of the play classes. After the program has ended, the software would go to the Pay attention mode, and you may pause each audio anytime; you can even record a custom relaxing sound.

4. Lullabytes

This lovely iPhone application to help children sleep is amazingly easy to navigate. It utilizes the thought of lullabies to assist the infant in sleeping. They have twelve piano music that you can select from and gets the option to add information; like the time a baby will take to drift off and the sleeping time.

Additionally, they have many sounds to eliminate the silence as the infant sleeps, specially when recently born. It detects the baby's wail and immediately has the sounds.

5. Novel Effect

Novel Effect is a superb iPhone application to help children sleep, and it's over one million downloads that shows it's well-liked by mothers. The application is exclusive and has music as you narrate stories to the infant, similar to films. It takes on original music as well as sound files that match particular kids' books.

The software gives you to choose a book and begin reading it to your child. The app's tone of voice acknowledgement system will know your situation in the storyplot and play music appropriately to own perfect music results. Through the app, you can gain access to books like 'Kitty in the Hat' and 'Where in fact the Crazy Things Are'.

6. Nighty Night

This application has been created by Heidi Wittlinger, who's an animator and illustrator and was simply nominated for an Oscar award; it really is a narrated tale iphone app about the whereabouts and activities of barnyard pets after lights venture out. Your child will see pets drift off in their habitat, assisting these to do the same.

The application costs $3. 99, which really is a low priced for a good iPhone application to help children sleep.

7. Sleepy Sounds

Sleepy Sounds can be an iPhone application that plays relaxing nature sounds and lullabies on the loop while displaying an animated mobile that lightens up the area of your son or daughter. This application is another free iPhone application to help children sleep.

8. Sleepy Hero

This iphone app gives you available summary of sounds that are pre-recorded. You can even upload your own tales, music, and nursery rhymes. Whenever your child starts to cry, the application reacts by playing your custom selection. The application is an excellent iPhone application to help children sleep but costs $2. 78.

In conclusion; if you're sick and tired of hearing your

child cry in the middle of the night, the other of these applications can help you. You won't have to awaken to soothe the infant to sleep as the application will do the task for you. Download an iPhone application to help children sleep.

Chapter 11

How Babies Adapt to Timezone Changes

Getting the baby on any semblance of a standard sleep schedule can frequently be beyond challenging! but , after you have finally founded a routine, as well as your baby is on the schedule and also sleeping, you don't want to wreck havoc on it! You routine your dinner programs around it, get back after supper with friends much sooner than normal, and prevent scheduling sessions during naptime!

However, there are a few changes that people can't avoid: 'time changes!' Whether it's fall or springtime and the clocks are continual or backward by one hour or you've planned to go to someplace in a different time area, just considering these changes and assisting your baby adapt to time change distinctions can be nerve-wrecking! You don't want to screw up a very important thing and disturb your baby's timetable. Below, we have some tips which you can use to help your child adapt to time change distinctions.

Helping Your Child Adapt to Daylight Savings Time

Whenever we "fall back again" or "springtime forward, " we must adapt our clocks one hour. If you don't want your child to be up extra early, be very cranky and fussy during the night, and you need to be faraway from their normal regular for a couple of days, or weeks; following change, there are few strategies you can test in the times before and pursuing Daylight Cost savings Time.

Build a Dark Space For Sleep

As a grown-up, you can tell yourself that it's time to visit bed, or enjoy getting a supplementary hour of sleep in the fall. You can't simply show these exact things to your child and expect them to check out your wishes.

To help your child adapt to time change distinctions, you'll need to supply them with a dark space to sleep therefore the sun glowing through their home window doesn't wake them up. You are able to consider purchasing black-out drapes which will stop more light arriving through their home window than traditional drapes or a tone.

Gradually Move Your Baby's Bedtime

Rather than expecting your child to immediately adjust to their bedtime and wake time changing by a complete hour in one day to another, gradually change your baby's schedule.

Through the week before Daylight Savings Time, slowly move your baby's bedtime forward or backwards by a few momemts every day depending about how enough time will be changing. This can help your baby adapt to time change variances more steadily.

Keep Your Child up Just a little Longer

Depending on your child, maintaining your baby up simply a few extra minutes (or placing them down a few momemts early) on the night time of Daylight Savings Time, may be adequate to help your child adapt to time change differences.

You might be in a position to move their bedtime by twenty or thirty minutes to help them adapt to enough time change. However , not absolutely all babies will be the same, which won't work for any babies.

Wait a few moment before getting the baby each day

If on the morning hours of Daylight Cost savings Time, your child wakes up one hour early (at the same time as their normal wake time), wait around a few momemts prior to going to their room to wake them up.

If you hurry right directly into their rooms as of this early hour, it's possible that their sleep schedule will adapt to the new, earlier awaken time. Waiting a little can help your child adapt to time change distinctions and sleep better soon!

Follow Your Normal Timetable and Routine

You might have a few rough times with a cranky or fussy baby, but it's important to stick to the schedule and regimen you want your child to check out. Help your child modify to time change variations by keeping a steady schedule and placing them down for naps and bedtime at when you used prior to the time change.

Helping Your Child Adjust to Planning a trip to a Different Time Zone

When you happen to be in a fresh time area, it may also be challenging for your child to adjust. If the time is only going to be one hour different or ten hours different, it can still impact your baby.

There are a few strategies you can test to ease the consequences of that time period change on your child.

Start Shifting to the brand new Time before Your

Trip Begins

In the times or weeks before your trip, slowly modify your child's schedule so that it is more based on the new time zone you'll be visiting. Try pressing their bedtime forwards or backwards by ten or a quarter-hour per day until these are nearer to the timetable you'll want these to be on. This can help your baby adapt to time change distinctions associated with planing a trip to a fresh destination.

Look for a Red-Eye Flight

If it's possible, look for a red-eye air travel, particularly if you are planing a trip to a time area that is multiple hours not the same as your home time; your child is going to be exhausted and prepared to sleep on the airplane which can help your child adapt to time changes distinctions in the new time area you'll be going to.

Show Patience and Reassure Your Child

Think about how exactly you feel if you are jet-lagged from planing a trip to a fresh time zone, are you feeling off and in a fog? Visualize how your child must be feeling. Below are a few actions you can take to help your child adapt to time change distinctions:

✓ Remain patient and understanding

✓ Reassure your child that everything is OK

✓ Offer a lot of snuggles, hugs, and kisses to help your child feel safe and loved

✓ Model sticking with your normal routines

It could be challenging for an infant to change to time change variations in their routines. The change with time, even only if one hour, can toss their routine up in the air and leave them sense exhausted, cranky, and puzzled. Hopefully, a few of the recommendations we've offered in this specific article will help you to help your child change to time change variances without either of you experiencing the change!

Chapter 12

8 Ideas to Bring Your Child to Work and Stay Productive

It has been said again and again that there's no chance that ladies can own it all; that expecting and an effective career is a dream. As it happens that these are simply just opinions which have a minor basis. The complete notion of "leave the area when you have to change a diaper" is a hoax. Yes, you could have an incredible profession but still experience your child's milestones. In case your maternity leave is going to eliminate and you are feeling guilty about departing your baby, you can consider taking your child to work.

So, exactly what does it take to remain productive in your place of work while caring for your child?

All you have to do is plan, support and strategize.

Tips when planning on taking your child to any office

Here's how to ace this fantastic plan of experiencing your baby at work.

1 . Find out your company's policies

Self-employed moms don't need to check up on the policies since it is their enterprise plus they can established the guidelines. However, employed moms must give this consideration. Understand the company's plan in relation to taking your child to work; if the plan will not allow, speak to your company and observe how you could work things out. Going to work with your child unannounced is dangerous and it might lead to the increased loss of your job.

2 . Involve your partner

It really is normal to feel just like you have small time with your baby. Take extreme care and don't be over possessive about any of it because you may finish up doing everything by yourself, yet your lover is ready to chip in. Tell them what you will like assist with. For instance, you may be pleased to take your child to work interchangeably, that way, you can convenience the strain and the kid will feel the love of both parents.

3. Co-worker supervisor support

Among the factors that regulate how successful taking baby to work will be is the support you obtain from your supervisor and co-workers. You must determine this before making a decision on taking your child to any office. Interview them without always disclosing what your plan is. Once you're sure that they might not actually mind you bringing your child to work, you can inquire further what they've experienced about your idea. Sometimes co-workers aren't open to the idea but as time passes they warm-up, and the changeover is effortless.

4. Require help

You aren't guaranteed that taking your child to work will continue to work out flawlessly all-day and every day. So , you should find a person who will back you up again if you are unavailable. Ask one of your co-workers to stand set for you when you can't be with the infant because you need to focus on an immediate matter at work. Using a pre-organized set up ensures that there is no need downtime at the job and that you will get to keep your task to the finish. Team work is of the substance.

5. Carry all the requirements

Taking your child to work will be easier when you yourself have the proper tools. Possessing a carrier is vital as it'll make it easier that you should carry your son or daughter around any office as you are printing documents or perform other minor jobs. Depending on the age group, you might reap the benefits of having some playthings too, consider the elements when packaging your essentials. Picture the most severe case situation, such as what would happen if the air conditioning equipment halted working and you are in the center of summer.

Other essential items include:

✓ Bibs

- ✓ Extra clothes

- ✓ Diapers

- ✓ Wipes

- ✓ Burp Cloths

6. When the infant sleeps, use enough time wisely

Whether your son or daughter is asleep or awake, you should focus on being at your very best within the task environment. When taking your child to work, you should concentrate on making use of your time productively. You are able to group your jobs into the ones that require maximum attention and the ones that don't. Whenever your baby is sleeping, you are able to do the high-attention jobs and find yourself the low-attention responsibilities whenever your child is awake.

7. Make good use of the lunch time break

Whether you are permitted to break for one hour or thirty minutes, how you have this time around will help simplicity of the strain of taking your child to any office.

In the event that you haven't gotten sufficient time for you to sleep, this is your chance at napping without concern with judgment. You can even utilize this chance to unwind and play with your baby. When you have not given the kid, this is a great chance to do so.

8. Recognize that this is temporary

When the stresses of taking your child to work meet up with you, understand that this is a short-term arrangement. Soon, they'll be ready for college, and you'll not need to bring them daily. So, enjoy your precious occasions of taking your child to any office when you still can.

You could have it all!

An operating mom realizes that she actually is a good parent because of her job rather than regardless of it. Research has it that a working mom who considers taking her baby to work is proficient, content and socially linked. With all the current benefits that taking your child to any office draws in, you haven't any reason never to own it all!

Chapter 13

Childhood Sleep Apnea: 8 Signs or symptoms

When you have heard your son or daughter snore or he/she seems like he/she is not sleeping well, you might wonder, does your son or daughter have sleep apnea? Sleep apnea may appear just like a condition that impacts the elderly, but sleep apnea in children is very real and can result in a variety of mental, physical and sociable problems. When questioning if your son or daughter has sleep apnea, it seems sensible to understand precisely what sleep apnea in children is.

What is Sleep Apnea in Children?

Sleep apnea is an ailment where the person stops respiration at certain factors while asleep. This typically is really because there is certainly something blocking top of the airway. This form of sleep apnea is named obstructive sleep apnea.

Sleep apnea in children can cause interrupted sleep. When you stop respiration, even momentarily, the air levels in the torso drop, which disrupt the sleep cycle. This helps it be more challenging for someone experiencing sleep apnea to obtain a sleepful night's sleep. If neglected, sleep apnea in children can cause behavior, learning, center and development problems.

Causes of Sleep Apnea in Children

It really is normal for the muscles to relax as you sleep. If the muscles in the rear of the neck relax too much, the airway can collapse. They are the muscles accountable for keeping the airway open up, so when they become excessively calm it causes trouble deep breathing. In people with enlarged adenoids or tonsils, the blockage can be even more serious.

There are a number of things that can cause sleep apnea in children. They include carrying excess fat, a family background of sleep apnea, a sizable tongue, this may fall back again and build a blockage in the airway, framework issues in the neck, jaw or mouth area that induce a slim airway, or other medical ailments such as cerebral palsy or Down symptoms.

Inhaling and exhaling through the mouth area may indicate your son or daughter is experiencing or reaches threat of developing sleep apnea. Humans are made to inhale through their noses, so mouth area deep breathing indicates something is incorrect. If the nose passages are constricted, credited to allergy symptoms, for example , your son or daughter may start deep breathing through his mouth area. When deep breathing through the mouth area, the jaw muscles occur a relaxed condition and can result in weakness in the muscles of the mouth area and throat, this may lead to sleep apnea in children.

Symptoms of Sleep Apnea in Children

Real sleep apnea spells often occur without the average person realizing it. When you stop respiration, the air level in the torso drops quickly and the skin tightens and level rises; that is an indicator for the mind to wake you up. You awaken to inhale and get back to sleep so quickly you don't realize you were awake. This pattern repeats itself at night time, avoiding you from possessing a sleepful, deep sleep.

In the event that you hear your son or daughter snoring, particularly with snorts, pauses or gasps, he might be experiencing sleep apnea shows. Sleepless sleep, and sleeping in unusual positions are also indications of sleep apnea in children. Heavy deep breathing, daytime sleepiness, night time terrors, sleepwalking, and bedwetting can all also indicate sleep apnea in children.

In the event that you notice your son or daughter milling his teeth, you might investigate whether he's suffering from sleep apnea. If the smooth tissues behind the neck are obstructing the airway, milling or clenching one's teeth may be considered an indication that your body is wanting to open up the airway. Milling and clenching your tooth tightens in the tongue and jaw muscles and can help start the airway.

Because your son or daughter is not obtaining a good night's sleep, you might have trouble waking them up each day. They may drift off, be hyperactive, and also have trouble focusing throughout the day. These symptoms make a difference in college performance, and business lead to the instructor thinking they have ADHD or other learning issues.

Diagnosing Sleep Apnea in Children

If your son or daughter is a sleepless sleeper, snores, falls asleep throughout the day or exhibits other signs of sleep apnea, you might wonder, does your son or daughter have sleep apnea? It's important to seek advice from with your child's pediatrician about your concerns. He might want to send your son or daughter to an expert who may choose to perform a sleep study.

Sleep studies are accustomed to diagnose sleep problems, including sleep apnea in children. Your son or daughter should spend the night time in a sleep center to endure the sleep research. Sleep studies are accustomed to measure snoring and other sounds, blood air, and skin tightening and levels, body actions and positions, heartrate, eye actions, brain waves, and inhaling and exhaling patterns.

Treatment For Sleep Apnea in Children

There are a number of treatments designed for sleep apnea. They include:

- ✓ Observation
- ✓ Surgery
- ✓ CPAP
- ✓ Mouthguard
- ✓ Weight Loss

If the sleep apnea is relatively moderate, rather than interfering with your child's standard of living, your doctor might want to monitor symptoms for some time, before making a decision on cure. If the reason for sleep apnea is enlarged, tonsils or adenoids, your physician may refer your son or daughter to a ear, nose, and neck specialist. The ENT may choose to remove either the tonsils, adenoids or both. These methods may be all that's needed is to get rid of the sleep apnea.

Your doctor might want your son or daughter to use continuous positive airway pressure therapy. CPAP counseling requires your son or daughter to wear a face mask covering the nasal area or/and mouth while asleep. The mask links to a machine that uses air to keep carefully the airways open.

Based on your child's age group and the reason behind sleep apnea, he might have the ability to wear a mouthguard during sleep to prevent shows of sleep apnea. These mouthguards generally work best on teenagers but can be utilized on children as young as six.

If your physician believes that weight may be the reason contributing factor to your child's sleep apnea, she/he will probably recommend lifestyle and diet changes to aid safe weight loss. Sometimes achieving a wholesome weight will do to put an end to shows of sleep apnea.

Complications of Sleep Apnea

When wondering if your son or daughter have sleep apnea, you might be tempted to place off diagnostics. Sleep studies, although pain-free and safe, tend to be scary to small children. It's important to comprehend that snoring is definitely not something safe. You should speak to your pediatrician to access underneath the snoring concern before it influences your child.

Studies claim that snoring, even though not linked with sleep apnea, can result in a variety of medical issues in children. Knowing that, it's important to research and treat snoring and sleep issues.

Sleep apnea is considered to increase fragmentation in sleep. This means your body is continually switching in one sleep stage to some other. This change between lighter and heavier sleep cycles don't allow your son or daughter to get the long amount of deep sleepful sleep they need.

Children who have sleep apnea may experience the symptoms comparable to adults, when they are drowsy throughout the day, however they are just likely to react to this insomnia by developing public problems, having difficulty attending to, becoming hyper, or experiencing intervals of unhappiness or nervousness. Children who don't sleep well will perform badly on memory space and learning assessments.

Children who experience sleep apnea not only develop emotional and mental symptoms, they can experience physical problems as well. Disruption of deep sleep can hinder hormone secretion, including growth hormones. With less growth hormones available, normal development patterns can be adversely affected.

As you can plainly see, sleep apnea can result in a variety of medical issues. If you're wondering if your son or daughter have sleep apnea, it's important to get answers. If you were to think your son or daughter may be experiencing sleep apnea, you should have a scheduled appointment with your pediatrician to go over your concerns.

Chapter 14

Reasons why Your Child won't Laugh or be Happy

Parents live for those giggles and smiles their infants give, so noticing that your child isn't happy could be disconcerting.

The next information will educate you on infants and laughter so you know very well what steps to take if your child isn't happy.

When Your Baby Start to Laugh?

The very first thing that needs to be addressed is the likelihood that your child isn't laughing due to the fact it isn't the right time. Yes, it holds true that most infants commence to chuckle when they reach ninety days, but there are a few who take up to four weeks to elegance you using their laughter.

It will also be remarked that your child is still understanding how to control the tongue and mouth area.

Which means that even though you hear your child laugh once, it does not mean you will hear it again.

Try to show patience because your little baby might possibly not have a good understanding on his/her capability to laugh at this time. Give your son or daughter time before jumping to the final outcome that your child isn't happy or your child isn't laughing in any way.

It might be possible a baby who isn't happy or an infant who isn't laughing just requires a little force in the right path, and you could assist with that.

Ideas to Help Your Child Laugh

Your child may be going for a while due to the fact they're not engaged. Make an effort to create a host to help your son or daughter laugh. There are many actions you can take, like ensuring your child is comfortable, given, and burped if needed.

Taking these steps means that your infant is preparing to have fun. If an infant is unhappy, the infant isn't laughing any time in the future. Listed below are some actions you can take to attempt to make your son or daughter have fun:

Auditory Oddities: Some respond easier to funny appears like squeaks or popping sounds, so try those.

Video games: Peek-a-boo and other fun video games might do just fine.

Strange Feelings: Yes, your child may need to experience things such as blowing on their skin or light tickling to giggle.

Those that see their baby make a variety of joyful noises like chirps, coos, or gurgles may not need to worry. The giggle is coming. Your child just hasn't understood how to vocalize a laughter properly, so give your son or daughter some time.

It will also be remarked that there is certainly any such thing as a significant disposition. You almost certainly have met some individuals with "old souls. "

An infant with a significant disposition is not really a baby who isn't happy or an infant who isn't laughing because something is incorrect; it may be you need to know who your child is. Your little angel will have fun about something, but it'll simply take her or him a little much longer to find that perfect minute.

Perhaps your child must hear other activities you never have tried, like the sound of velcro or the sound of the zipper closing or opening.

It might be just a little strange, but there are infants whose love of life is so peculiar that you will be have to to obtain a little creativity to encourage them to have fun. Usually do not fret, all you have to use is the internet plus some patience.

When for Anyone Who is Concerned?

It might be nice to state that all infants will laugh sooner or later, but the the truth is that sometimes an infant isn't happy for grounds. Yes, sometimes a parent's concern can be described away, but periodically a parent understands there's a reason an infant isn't laughing.

One of the most clear signs that your child isn't happy or your child isn't laughing for grounds is if your son or daughter has missed other common milestones.

A baby is meant going to a few milestones as time progresses, which lets you know that your little angel is really as healthy as they might be, however, many children have developmental issues. An infant who isn't happy or an infant who isn't laughing can be considered an indication of trouble if you place other activities, like your child not spontaneously smiling.

Children are likely to smile randomly by four weeks old. Your little angel is also said to be in a position to follow things active for him or her with the eye.

Your child should recognize faces by four months and

have a genuine curiosity about playing with other people. As stated before, your child also needs to be making babbling or cooing noises by now.

It's important that you observe these and other developmental milestones that your son or daughter hasn't hit yet, even though she or he must have. All of this information is likely to be helpful when you take your child to see a medical expert to be properly diagnosed.

Other Reasons Your Child isn't Laughing

There may be a significant underlying issue with your little baby, and you will need to ensure your physician identifies why your child isn't happy. Trust your intuition upon this because dealing with what is correct with your son or daughter early usually makes things better for everybody.

An infant who isn't happy might not be happy because

she or he could be experiencing a variety of issues, like hearing problems.

Much of just what a baby does depends upon your baby's ability to imitate, figure out how to make sounds you make, and pay attention to just how sounds happen. Just a little cherub who's having troubles hearing or cannot listen to in any way will never be able to strike this milestone or a few of the others.

An infant who isn't laughing could also have developmental issues because she or he is not subjected to many noises or words. Failing woefully to provide enough arousal may lead to an infant who isn't happy and nobody wants that.

There are a great number of reasons a parent may have trouble providing a stimulating environment; for example, you may be working several job, perhaps you have other kids to be concerned about.

You are able to address this in several ways; for example, you can transform your plan around to provide your baby additional time. Parents can also hire professional babysitters who learn how to help a kid develop by speaking with the child a bit more and dedicating time.

No matter the reason why, figuring out the proceedings with an infant who isn't laughing or an infant who isn't happy should help your physician create an action plan.

Another reason your child isn't laughing could be associated with autism. This is certainly something no mother or father wants to assume, but the the truth is that autism proceeds to rise in america, making this risk a lot more real.

Having the ability to diagnose this issue early should help you so you understand how you will increase your child effectively. Listed below are some indicators that may be letting you know your child has autism:

- ✓ Joyful sounds aren't present, such as cooing or chirping.

- ✓ Vision contact may be poor or nonexistent.

- ✓ Severe speech delays may start to show.

- ✓ Your child may develop extreme intesleep in a single thing at the same time.

- ✓ Several instances where your child displays

unusual reactions to sounds, tastes, sights, touch, or smells.

There is absolutely no doubt that seeing a few of these signs will cause you to feel anxious or scared; that is your son or daughter! You want the most effective for her or him, so that it is alright to have these types of emotions, but be sure you concentrate on his/her wellbeing.

You are heading to want to write down these additional signs and some other abnormal behavior which means that your doctor will help you move to the next step.

Hopefully, the information in this book will help you figure out the next steps or cause you to feel more relaxed because you have a firmer grasp on how to proceed for your child. Remember, there is absolutely no pity in requesting help anytime since it really does have a village to improve a happy and healthy baby.

Chapter 15

Reasons For Your Child's Tiredness

As a parent, it is only practical to create a host that facilitates medical protection and well-being of your son or daughter. That is why it's so important to be an attentive mother or father. In the event that you notice something that's uncommon or off, it's your responsibility to handle and rectify the problem.

With regards to parenting in the first years, it's not unusual for the kid to perform circles round the parent. Most parents do their finest to survive on a couple of hours of sleep and plenty of espresso. However, when you are ready and when you're operating circles around your son or daughter, something is off.

Which means that your son or daughter is always tired, which should raise a few pre-determined questions. A kid shouldn't maintain circumstances of total lethargy on a regular basis. If you've pointed out that your son or daughter is always exhausted, understand that there's a way to treat it. Have a look at the next reasons that can indicate why your son or daughter is always exhausted. Consider implementing the next solutions as well.

Reasons why your son or daughter is always tired:

1. Your son or daughter isn't getting enough sleep.

While you will find loads of parents who can't await bedtime, there are certainly others who allow their children to remain up all night. This isn't a good idea. It's very important for a kid to get their sleep in order to have the power to function the next day. Plus, when they're in that critical developmental period, their physiques need the chance to recharge.

A whole lot of development spurts happen during years as a child. This may be the key reason why parents think the youngster is always exhausted. In the end, it's not unusual for a kid to develop a few ins within a couple of months. When you allow your son or daughter to remain until the wee hours of the morning hours, this will have a primary effect on their capability to be alert and concentrated during the day.

To be able to rectify this example, it could be challenging to try a youthful bedtime with the cool turkey method. Instead, help your son or daughter work their way up to a youthful bedtime. If indeed they tend to blow wind down by midnight, begin to shoot for 11pm. Every night, ensure that you bump enough time back a quarter-hour.

Do your very best to avoid overstimulation before bedtime. When you have a young child, it's pretty good to shoot for 7 or 8pm as their new bedtime. You will find loads of studies that show the way the quality of sleep increases whenever a person reaches bed before midnight.

Plus, when you put your son or daughter in bed, this means that you'll have the ability to have a youthful bedtime yourself. Use a complete fourteen days to focus on moving the bedtime plan; as you think to do it earlier, you can test different strategies to trick your son or daughter into thinking it's later than it really is.

Blackout drapes make the area seem to be pitch-black. Even though it's 8 pm but still shiny outside, you may use the blackout drapes and go out in their bedroom until it's time for you to go down.

2 . Your child's dietary practices need improvement.

If you have a tendency to feed your son or daughter plenty of sugar-packed cereals, desserts and goodies, your son or daughter isn't getting the nutrition they have to support their body. Although it might seem to be simpler to feed your son or daughter fast food due to a busy schedule, recognize that this does anything to gas their body's dependence on energy.

Instead, start providing healthy foods on a constant basis. Whenever your child is always exhausted, be sure they're eating at breakfast time constantly as it's one of the most crucial meals of your day. Understand that it's insufficient to relish an instant pop-tart or instant waffle. Rather than cereals filled with sugars and bleached flour, consider attempting oatmeal with fruit. Scrambled eggs, toast and a green smoothie make a great power breakfast time combination.

Do your very best to incorporate fruits & vegetables atlanta divorce attorneys meal. For snack foods, try apple pieces rather than pudding. Rather than salty potato chips, try carrots with hummus. Supper might add a part salad for maximum nourishment. It's also a good idea to ensure your son or daughter receives their daily vitamin supplements.

Purchase vitamins in gummy or chewable form to boost the probability of intake. Remove sodas and juices with a great deal of sugars. Your child will receive a sugar spike, but they'll finish up crashing. If your son or daughter is always exhausted, a sugar spike and crash will be the last things you want them to see.

Instead, it's smart to incorporate more drinking water in to the regimen. If your son or daughter prefers some taste, it's okay to include a few lemon pieces and some strawberries to flavor. Research your facts to discover the suggested amount of sugars your son or daughter can have in a single day. Researchers have a tendency to share that quantity in grams.

Once you're clear on the total amount, always browse the brands. Two mugs of soda pop could easily go beyond a given amount when you're not attending to.

3. Your child's plan is too frantic.

As a mother or father, it only is practical so that you can ensure that your child has a packed plan. In the end, if they're not emotionally activated and challenged, you're not providing the best educational experience on their behalf. Although it is important to ensure your son or daughter remains occupied and emotionally stimulated, you'll be able to overschedule them.

If they're getting up early each day for daycare or college, they need to sit through a complete day in the class. Then, if you've planned after-school activities on their behalf, this involves more energy. This is also true if the actions are physical ones like going swimming, gymnastics and golf ball.

Instead, consider dialing back again on their day to day activities. If your son or daughter is always exhausted, provide them with more margin to relax. There are many parents who indicates what their children up for after-school activities since it keeps the kids occupied until they complete the task day. However, rather than signing your son or daughter up for just one more afterschool activity, consider finding a babysitter.

The babysitter can pick your son or daughter up after school. After they get back, the babysitter makes it possible for the child to consider a day nap before it's time to begin homework. That one change might make a significant difference in a child's capability to recharge and feel more alert throughout the standard day.

You'll be able to overstimulate your son or daughter. While it's completely noble and honorable to ensure your son or daughter is subjected to new principles, new friends and new encounters, it will never come at the trouble of their health. Create a relationship with your child's instructor.

If the teacher asks why your son or daughter is tired, be honest about the many problems you're taking a look at. Most educators have observed at least one young child appears to be more lethargic than others; because of this, they could have their own answers to offer.

4. Your son or daughter isn't getting quality sleep.

Finally, when you're examining the many reasons why your son or daughter is tired, it's important to consider their sleep regimen. If your son or daughter gets to bed promptly, but they're sleepless in the bed, they're heading to be exhausted during the day.

That is why it's such a wise idea for parents to implement a sleep regimen that's constant and practical. Whenever your child is always exhausted because of having less quality sleep, you'll desire to be intentional about creating a host that invites optimal sleep. Utilize blackout drapes to make a dark room.

Get rid of the nightlight if that stimulates overstimulation. A audio machine works for most children. Whether you utilize white noise, sea noises or rainfosleep noises, consider a sleep software or audio machine that delivers sleep. When it's time for you to have a nighttime shower, use soaps and creams with lavender.

Lavender has a relaxing effect. Consider investing in a diffuser. Fill up the diffuser with essential natural oils like eucalyptus and lavender. Both natural oils are recognized to help with sleep as well. Make certain the home remains peaceful once it's time for bed.

In the event where your son or daughter is always tired, you'll want to ensure that their dinner is nutritious enough to satiate. If your son or daughter will be in bed with an annoyed tummy, this will likely affect their capability to sleep deeply. Whenever a child is always exhausted, it's a good idea to provide them a bedtime drink.

Warm-up a glass of soy dairy or almond dairy. Put in a chamomile tea handbag to the dairy. Allow it boil. Once it cools down, let your son or daughter drink the warm dairy. This mixture can do miracles for a child's capability to drift off to a peaceful and deep sleep.

Conclusively; to be able to get clear on the explanations why, consider implementing a trial-and-error period. As you take into account various solutions, don't hesitate to get specialists included. Once you take your son or daughter to their principal care doctor for a typical check-up, don't ignore to bring this matter up.

Be immediate in asking them how come your child exhausted. The doctor typically sees various problems on a regular basis. Therefore, they'd have answers to offer from a medical standpoint. The same concept pertains to a nutritionist. Look for a nutritionist who could probably help you realize why your son or daughter is tired on a regular basis.

Once you consider these four areas and seek advice from the assistance of doctors, you ought to be in a position to get a remedy to your question. Because of this, your child are certain to get more sleep.

Chapter 16

7 Signs that Show Your Child is too old for Naps

Napping can be an important part of your child's schedule. You may question, *is your son or daughter too old to nap?* but that's not a straightforward question. Children need enough sleep to be able to grow and find out properly. Insomnia can also make your son or daughter fussy and hard to be friends with. As your child ages, her sleep needs changes. Before very long, you have a kid too old to nap.

Signs of a Child too Old to Nap

- Resists napping or bedtime

- Generally maintains a positive attitude each day, with few ups or downs

- Gets up easily each day, ready to begin the day

When is a Child too Old to Nap?

There is nobody age which means your kids is preparing to drop naps. Generally, children start falling their naps between the age group of three and five. Don't take this as a difficult and fast guideline, some children gladly quit their naps at two years of age, while some cling to the nap when these are entering kindergarten.

Napping or not napping is not really a definitive thing. While your son or daughter transitions to keeping up all day long, he/she may nap some times rather than nap on others. It is highly recommended to take a versatile attitude during this time period. Fighting to keep carefully the nap or cease can make the changeover worse than it requires to be.

Sleep Needs by Age

It's important to remember there is certainly nobody's point for a kid too old to nap. Each young one is specific, and the procedure of shedding the nap is steady. In general, small children need twelve to fourteen hours of sleep each night, and can probably sleep. Preschoolers need between eleven and twelve hours of sleep each night, plus some will get a few of that sleep in an evening nap, while some won't need to have a nap.

How to Recognize a Child too Old to Nap

If your son or daughter skips the casual nap that will not indicate he/she is prepared to quit his/her naps. More important is how the child reacts to the lack of nap. If your child dozes off later in the day or falls asleep once you put him/her in the automobile, she doesn't appear to be a kid too old to nap. Don't let these past due afternoon kitty naps replace a normal nap. Doing this makes it more challenging to get your child to nap during intercourse with your spouse at night.

If your son or daughter starts to withstand naptime, let him/her achieve this and observe how he/she acts. If your child makes it to bedtime without having to be excessively grumpy or psychological, your son or daughter may be too old to nap. If your child resists the nap but falls aside later in your day, your son or daughter isn't too old to nap.

Your Son or Daughter doesn't know best

It's quite common for children to combat to sleep before they will be ready to cease. This really is an extremely normal part of your child's development. It doesn't have anything regarding their physical maturity, rather it is due to cognitive maturity which makes your son or daughter want more control and autonomy. Physical maturity is exactly what separates a kid too old to nap to one who feels she is.

Despite the fact that this is a properly normal stage in your child's development, it doesn't mean you are going along with it. A kid too old to nap will be sleepless in his/her room during naptime, but a kid seeking to abandon naptime before actually ready can form behavioral issues. Allowing your kid to stop nap will lead to cranky behavior, hyperactivity, and other problems.

To encourage your son or daughter to nap, it could help to change in the nap schedule. Try seat with him/her and speak softly when you rub their back; let your kid know he/she doesn't have to sleep, just lay silently for some time. A good child too old to nap will love this time around, and if your son or daughter isn't too old to nap, laying silently for a few moments is usually all it requires on his/her behalf to drift off.

Be Flexible

While your son or daughter is moving from napping to staying up all day long, the normal program may need to pass the wayside. Some times she may nap, other times she might not. You might find moving the bedtime up to a youthful hour will benefit both of you on times she doesn't nap. Getting her before she becomes worn out and has a meltdown is effective for you both. Your son or daughter probably must sleep between 10 and 12 hours to feel her best.

Throughout that difficult change time, consider allowing go of the thought of a nap so long as your son or daughter agrees for some quiet time. Placing your son or daughter in her room with some silent playthings or books to amuse herself can be considered a good changeover to nap-free times. If your son or daughter is preparing to quit the naps, you can both get just a little break throughout the day. If she still needs the nap, she'll probably drift off in this quiet time.

Make an Effort to Maintain a Routine

Although it is normal for naptime to come and go in this transition period, it's important to work against some regularity. If you were to think your kid is preparing to quit naps, move bedtime back again a little so she actually is getting more sleep at night. If you don't believe your son or daughter is too old for naps, continue steadily to demand she spends time laying silently during intercourse at naptime.

Chapter 17

What to do whenever a Baby Sleeps with their Eyes Open

Having a fresh baby can be stressful because new mothers aren't always ready for the life span lessons that parenting shows them. Although it is wishful considering to think that you are this glorious fountain of knowledge who will have the ability to quickly solve any issue that your son or daughter faces, it requires lots of time to be always a supermom.

Among the strange occurrences that any new mom might face is walking to their baby's room and viewing an empty glassy-eyed stare on the child's frozen face. The savvy mother will know never to wake the kid because at least he seems relaxed and happy.

A less experienced mom may begin making jokes at how dazed their baby looks. Let's discuss this safe baby behavior of the freezing sleep stare in more detail below.

Although new and potential parents may haven't heard,

since it is seldom discussed, it is totally safe and normal *whenever a baby sleeps with their eyes open up. The trait is named **nocturnal lagophthalmos** in medical journals.* This problem can even happen in people but is known as normal and unremarkable whenever a baby sleeps using their eye open up.

Adults are recognized to stay in a hypnagogic condition before and after sleep if they're tired. This way, they could be thinking and hallucinating whilst they may be awake. Their eyelids may be heavy, as they nod off and move around in and out of awareness.

People in a hypnagogic condition could also have spiritual visions and also delve deeper to their unconscious mind. A lot of the prophetesses and folks of historic times could actually make predictions by drugging themselves into such claims to write as though possessed by the spirits of the lifeless utilizing a technique called necromancy.

How to proceed whenever a Baby Sleeps with their Eye Opened

There is absolutely nothing that you'll require to do if your child sleeps using their eyes open if you don't observe that they suffer from dry and irritated eyes. It really is only in the rasleep situations that the disorder is triggered by birth flaws that have an effect on the newborn's eyelids. Most infants will outgrow this behavior.

If it annoys you, you can merely use your hands to gently manipulate their eyelids closed when they may be sleeping. It really is a sensitive balance for new moms to risk waking a colicky child and letting them earn the staring competition.

Why does my baby sleep with eye opened?

Could Rapid Eye Movement (R. E. M.) Sleep Be at fault?

The reason for **nocturnal lagophthalmos** in babies is not readily known. Researchers have never yet found any serious reasons to invest in a huge research about them. However, they presently believe they have something regarding the kind of sleep that influences infants.

Babies experience a longer time of Rapid Eye Movement (R. E. M.) sleep than adults. R. E. M. sleep is an activity that helps your brain reorganize its thoughts to be able to function better. It really is believed that individuals who are sleep deprived can form psychosis and other health issues because they never reach circumstances of REM sleep.

It may likewise have something regarding an undeveloped nervous system. It might take time for the spinal-cord to build up the reflexive impulse of shutting the eyes. Through the REM sleep of adults, the eyes are moving quickly everywhere. In infants, it looks similar too, they may be glassy-eyed and looking aimlessly into space.

It might be funny to think about them as cellphones downloading alien information and instructions for his or her developmental improvement. Eventually, you can wager that your child is certain to get that important update and start shutting the eye throughout the sleep cycle.

Does Nocturnal Lagophthalmos Occur in Adults?

Yes. It is really regarded as approved to infants through the DNA of their parents. In the event that you see your child sleeping using their eye open, you might ask somebody or friend to see whether additionally you sleep with your eye opened during the night. The REM sleep cycle most probably occurs ninety minutes after dozing off. The REM stage is well known for creating the fantasy cycles which might be a windowpane into our unconscious minds.

While an infant sleeping using their eye open up is no big deal, a grown-up who still sleeps with even one attention opened may be cause for alarm. The most common causes for nocturnal lagophthalmos in people are thyroid disorders, neurological disorders in the cosmetic nerves, and even specific types of tumors.

If you're experiencing these problems as a grown-up, you might not find out about it because you are within an unconscious fantasy state. Your lover may well not contemplate it if indeed they think you are just awake and looking into space throughout a concurrent sleep routine.

Putting an infant sleeping with an opened eyes to sleep

If you are putting your child to sleep, you should stay alert for the first ninety minutes roughly to find out if your baby starts to get into this trance-like condition. You may even want to be certain of them regularly to observe how they are suffering from it.

Although you ought not worry about any of it or walk out your way to improve an all natural behavior, you can provide yourself satisfaction that their eyes will retain moisture. For, in reality, a great deal of men and women suffer eyesight problems from looking at television sets and other displays because they don't blink their eye normally and can cause dryness and discomfort.

Chapter 18

Baby Sucks Thumb to Sleep-off

You've probably heard the horror tales surrounding infants sucking their thumbs to drift off. Their everlasting tooth comes into play at varying sides, or they could suck their thumbs for the others of their lives. Certainly, there is some truth to these tales, but is sucking the thumb to drift off something you should worry about?

The quick response to this question is *no and yes*. Let's start by talking about why your child has started sucking her/his thumb to drift off and whether there are any advantages to it.

Reasons for Sucking of Thumb

To get started with, don't stress it too much. As of this age group, everything infants see makes its way with their mouths. It truly is a matter of time before her thumb discovers its safe haven right inside her pie gap.

Comfort

Apart from sticking everything in their mouths, there are other reasons your child sucks his thumb to drift off, the most frequent reason is it conveniences him. Sucking is mainly natural urges your son or daughter has; whether sucking on the container or breastfeeding from his momma, he's most relaxed when suckling. It seems sensible that thumb sucking would provide a similar sense of serenity.

Other known reasons for thumb sucking

As your baby is continually subjected to new encounters and environments, sucking his thumb offers him ways to feel secure among all the newness. Along with comforting him/herself at bedtime or in new environments, there are many other reasons your child has considered thumb sucking. Included in these are:

✓ He might be hungry.

✓ He might be sleepy.

✓ He might be nervous or unsure of his environment.

✓ He might be bored.

What are the benefits to sucking the thumb to drift off?

One clear advantage whenever your baby sucks her thumb to drift off is that your child can self-soothe. Better still, she can get it done anywhere and anytime with no need for a pacifier. Perhaps have you ever tried to discover a pacifier at nighttime or underneath your handbag while shopping? Challenging.

What are some downfalls to sucking the thumb to drift off?

Weaning

One downfall whenever your baby sucks his thumb to drift off is that it could be difficult for your son or daughter to avoid. Unlike a pacifier, you are unable to take your child's thumb away. Later, we will discuss some very nice options to assist with weaning. Due to the products, I only know two different people who still suck their thumbs to drift off as adults.

Tooth and Speech

Another downfall whenever your baby sucks his thumb to drift off long-term, it can screw up the alignment of your child's long term teeth and even the roofing of his mouth area. You can not only be prepared to spend a little lot of money on orthodontics, however, many children will create a lisp from thumb sucking.

What is it possible to do?

Like we've said, don't be concerned too much. If your son or daughter continues to be very young, sucking his thumb won't hurt him/her. It's quite common for some children to avoid sucking their thumbs independently between age groups two and four.

Think about your child's thumb sucking style

One more thing to consider is that thumb sucking is not created similar. Which means that some children are more intense suckers while some passively keep their thumb in their mouths. An intense sucker will put more pressure on her behalf mouth and tooth which can cause more harm. In the event that you hear an audible popping audio when her thumb is taken off her mouth, you might have an intense sucker, and weaning early might be necessary.

Speak to your dentist

Your dentist is a superb resource to locating out if your son or daughter sucking her thumb to drift off is making a problem for budding teeth. It is strongly recommended that thumb sucking should stop before everlasting tooth start growing in. This can help to ensure that the habit won't affect your child's smile. Based on the American Teeth Association, most children start shedding their baby tooth and begin growing everlasting tooth around age group five or six.

When it's time for you to wean

Weaning can be especially problematic for a thumb sucker. While I asked my little girl why she sucked her thumb, she explained it experienced good inside. How was I heading to eliminate something that made her feel great inside? Fortunately, there are numerous products on the marketplace to help you with weaning whenever your child doesn't want to avoid sucking her thumb to drift off.

If your son or daughter simply isn't prepared to quit thumb sucking, you might like to get one of these thumb sucking glove. These gloves are constructed of plastic material and work through the elimination of suction with microscopic holes or vents. A kid can still put his thumb in his mouth area but is only going to have the ability to suck on air moving through the vents. The theory is that missing the suction, your son or daughter will see sucking his thumb less pleasant and eventually stop. One caveat of the method is that teenagers might be able to take away the glove.

Another solution to help you wean your thumb sucker is a particular type of toenail polish. You color it on your child's thumb (or any offending digit) toenail. Whenever your child places her thumb in her mouth area, she actually is greeted with a disgusting flavor. This technique works quickly if you don't have an ardent sucker who'll force through the flavor.

If the above mentioned methods been employed by, it could be smart to give a substitute to his thumb sucking. Since he probably uses his habit to comfort himself, it is effective that you can notice what sets off his thumb sucking (bedtime, new places, etc.) You can offer a little stuffed pet or a little blanket of these times.

The end of a time

In the long run, thumb sucking and the cessation from it is merely another part of life. You absolutely don't need to be concerned too much if your child uses his/her thumb to comfort him/herself. So long as your son or daughter has halted this habit before his long term teeth start growing in, you shouldn't have to be concerned about astronomical orthodontic expenses or impaired conversation.

Chapter 19

Important Foods to Avoid or Consume

When some moms have a baby, they worry that they need to completely overhaul their diet. Although it is important to consume healthier when pregnant, will this means that you have to state goodbye to your preferred foods? Even though you generally avoid processed foods, during pregnancy, it is a lot more important to ensure that your daily diet will be of advantage your child as well.

Your Daily Diet During Pregnancy

Your daily diet during pregnancy is focused on making sure your child gets the right nutrition. You're eating for just two now, so it's time to ensure your diet is really as baby-friendly as it can be. Some foods that might not have damaged you prior to getting pregnant may actually create a risk to your growing baby.

Do's or Don't: What Foods are Safe to Consume

Many moms want to keep to eating just how they did preceeding carrying a child. Based on each person's specific diet, this is totally fine or possibly dangerous. Using cases, there could be a few foods that you should scale back on or avoid completely for the period of you being pregnant. Continue reading for answers to the mostly asked questions about being pregnant and food.

May I Eat Sushi while Pregnant?

With regards to raw fish and pregnancy, main questions mothers ask their doctors are, " May I eat sushi while pregnant?" From a medical perspective, eating sushi while pregnant poses hardly any threat for you or your son or daughter. However, because of the fact that a lot of sushi is manufactured with raw seafood, it's important to ensure that the seafood in the sushi has been iced first if you are eating sushi while pregnant.

Likewise, when eating sushi while pregnant, you should attempt to limit your intake of raw fish. That is because of the fact that some organic fish includes small parasitic worms that can cause sickness and other medical issues.

In the event that you can't say no to eating sushi while pregnant, avoid the next types of sushi:

- ✓ Yellowfin tuna
- ✓ Horse mackerel
- ✓ Adult yellowtail
- ✓ Young yellowtail
- ✓ Swordfish
- ✓ Bluefin, yellowfin, bigeye
- ✓ Blue Marlin
- ✓ Albacore tuna
- ✓ Sea bass

If you really like eating sushi while pregnant, choosing vegetarian options like the California move is another way to work around potential dangers of consuming organic fish.

May I Eat Tuna While Pregnant?

If you're intesleeped in the health dangers of eating tuna while pregnant, it depends on the kind of tuna you take in, as well as how often you do eat it. Tuna, like all seafood includes traces of mercury, eating tuna while pregnant makes it possible for this mercury to enter the blood stream of both mother and the kid.

Moms eating tuna while pregnant will see that these degrees of mercury can negatively have an effect on their child's nervous system. So, if you're still wanting to know, " May I eat tuna while pregnant?", look into the FDA's suggestions below when eating tuna while pregnant:

✓ Limit you to ultimately twelve ounces of canned tuna.

✓ Limit you to ultimately six ounces of canned albacore or fresh tuna.

✓ Adhere to six ounces of fresh locally caught seafood.

In the event that you carefully monitor your cooked and canned tuna intake, eating tuna while pregnant shouldn't cause a problem.

May I Eat Crab While Pregnant?

In the event that you loved crab before you became pregnant, you're likely thinking to yourself, " May I eat crab while pregnant?" Just like some sea food can be harmful because of the degrees of mercury, it is right of you to question if eating crab while pregnant is dangerous.

With regards to sea food overall, eating crab is an excellent way to obtain vitamins D and A, as well as protein and omega-3 essential oil. Likewise, crab, like other sea food, aids in the attention and brain development of your son or daughter.

With regards to eating crab while pregnant, the FDA recommends that mothers adhere to prepared crab. Eating crab while pregnant will raise the mother's potential for developing food poisoning if the crab is organic. With imitation crab, eating crab while pregnant shouldn't cause a lot of a problem, so long as the imitation crab isn't followed by some other natural fish, you ought to be fine.

May I Eat Shrimp While Pregnant?

Shrimp is part of several well known recipes which is hard to avoid eating while pregnant if you're an enthusiast of fresh sea food. If you're concerned and thinking, "May I eat shrimp while pregnant?", the answer is yes.

While moms should limit their sea food intake and prevent high-mercury seafood, eating shrimp while pregnant is relatively safe. That is because of the fact that shrimp is classified as a low-mercury sea food. So long as the shrimp is fresh and prepared properly, mothers must have no issue when eating shrimp while pregnant.

Shrimp Benefits During Pregnancy

If you're excited to listen to the news headlines about eating shrimp while pregnant, retain in brain that you should still consume shrimp in moderate amounts. Adhere to smaller dosages of 340g every week. Apart from this sleepriction, there are several health advantages to eating shrimp:

- ✓ Shrimp is lower in fat.
- ✓ Shrimp is saturated in proteins and can promote fetal development.
- ✓ Every 100gm of your shrimp contains 1.8gm of iron.
- ✓ Shrimp is a great way to obtain omega-3.

May I Eat hot Canines while Pregnant?

Challenging various pregnancy cravings you'll have, hot dogs risk turning into one of your staples. Whether or not you regularly ate hot canines before being pregnant or you've lately obtained a craving on their behalf, it's smart to ask, " *May I eat hot canines while pregnant?* "

Eating hot pet dogs while pregnant isn't inherently harmful, but it will be is determined by the type of hot pet dogs you are eating. Ready-to-eat favorites like hot canines cause a risk for women that are pregnant because of the potential that they could contain parasites.

These cold-cut meat contain bacteria like listeria monocytogenes, which is why eating hot canines while pregnant is potentially dangerous. These bacterias can result in listeriosis, which make a difference both to the mom and the kid. In the even worse case situations, this bacterias can lead to premature delivery, disease, and miscarriage.

When eating hot canines while pregnant, take the time to properly increase temperature of these meats. Temperature will destroy the listeria monocytogenes, when hot canines are prepared sufficiently. Whether moms boil, microwave, or barbeque grill these canines, when thoroughly warmed, eating hot canines while pregnant should be properly fine.

May I Eat Sea Food while Pregnant?

With all that you now find out about crab, tuna, shrimp, and sushi, it's safe to state that the response to *"May I eat seafood while pregnant?"*, depends upon a number of factors.

Eating seafood while pregnant is an excellent way to get important nutrients and vitamins, however in limited quantities. As sea food includes essential omega-3 essential oil, it's very beneficial for moms to eat sea food frequently. However , due for some seafood's higher degrees of mercury, it extremely important for moms to watch what kind of sea food they eat, as well as how a lot of this sea food they eat.

Regarding to certain studies, eating seafood while pregnant is a significant element in how their babies develop. Moms that ate seafood 2-3 times a week throughout their being pregnant saw their infants reach certain developmental milestones faster than the kids of moms that didn't consume as much sea food.

What Seafood to consume While Pregnant

Do you like eating sea food? If you're at home or from the city and want to begin eating sea food while pregnant, try the next ideas:

- ✓ Grilled fish kabobs

- ✓ Mac-n-cheese with salmon, tuna, or lobster

- ✓ Shrimp stir-fry

- ✓ Seafood pasta

- ✓ Seafood sliders or burgers

✓ Seafood tacos.

If you're eating sea food while pregnant, keep these pointers at heart when you get the seafood to ensure it remains fresh:

✓ Choose the fresh seafood last so that it remains cool so long as possible.

✓ Thaw frozen seafood inside the refrigerator or in a sealed handbag with cool water.

As you take into account your daily diet during being pregnant, make sure to keep this guide about sea food, hot canines, and sushi at heart. No matter whatever cravings you might have, make sure to speak to a health care provider or dietitian in what foods will be best for your growing baby.

Chapter 20

Is Teeth Milling in Children Normal?

You imagine your little angel is sleeping peacefully during the night, but one night you hear it. It's an unmistakable, remarkably loud audio of teeth milling. If your child is milling the teeth, you may be worried. What's leading to it and how will you stop your son or daughter from milling their teeth?

Milling is Common

A great number of small children grind their teeth during the night, called "bruxism,"; this behavior typically starts at around four weeks old and can continue for a couple of years.

Some experts think that about three atlanta divorce attorneys' ten children grind their teeth. It's usually in impulse for some type of pain, but it generally isn't serious. If your child is milling his teeth, you aren't alone.

In adults, tooth grinding is generally a signal of stress or anxiety. If you're convinced that your child doesn't have almost as much to feel consumed with stress about as you need to do, you're right. You will find usually other reasons your that child is milling his teeth.

Reasons Your Child is Milling Teeth

Below are a few common things that could be leading to the nighttime sounds via your toddler's bedroom.

It's a Teeth or Teething Problem

In case your toddler's teeth hurt, she might respond by massaging them, like the way we rub and grind our very own teeth when they ache. She's most likely not even aware that she's carrying it out. Your child's teeth pain could be triggered by:

- ✓ Tooth that aren't fully aligned.
- ✓ New tooth growing in.
- ✓ A cracked tooth.

If your son or daughter is going right through teething

aches, he'll use the milling in an effort to sooth the pain. Generally, this is the reason why your child is milling his tooth. It's a reply to distress that helps her soothe herself.

When do you intervene?

The only time you should be concerned is if there's a broken or cracked teeth that may be leading to problems. If your child rubs his jaw frequently, that may be an indicator of teeth or jaw harm; if so, a trip to the dental professional will do.

How to proceed:

If your son or daughter is teething or working with improperly aligned tooth, then you don't need to be concerned. If your child is milling his tooth frequently and you see jaw massaging or other things that factors to an agonizing tooth problem, seek advice from your child's dental professional.

Something's Making Her Anxious

Although anxiety is usually the reason why people grind their teeth, it can occur to children as well. Some children are delicate to stress in the house. If there's been fighting or yelling inside your home, your child might feel pressure that inhibits her sleep. Others can feel annoyed with a change in regular, a fresh sibling or a fresh environment.

If your child is milling his teeth the night time before school, there could be something happening with a teacher or a fellow pupil that has upset him. Your very best approach is to discover what's creating this problem and find out if there's ways to place it to sleep.

How to proceed:

If you believe your baby is annoyed about something at home or at preschool, provide them with verbal and physical reassurance that everything is likely to be fine. Practice any relaxing rituals you have that normally helps him/her sleep.

It's important to help your children deal using their emotional concerns. If your child is milling his tooth now, a very important thing you can certainly do is intervene lightly. Stress-related teeth milling can continue into adolescence and adulthood if the foundation of the strain isn't resolved.

It Could have a Medical Cause

Certain medical ailments can cause teeth grinding in children. Included in these are cerebral palsy and hyperactivity. If your child is milling his tooth and it's related to a condition, speak to your doctor about ways to help your son or daughter. Some children also grind their tooth as a reply to queasy.

How to proceed:

If you're already monitoring your child's health, observe any indication that the milling is increasing the problem. Point out your concerns at the next pediatric visit, it's likely that there's nothing at all serious occurring, but it's always smart to make sure.

For Anyone who is worried that Your Child is Milling Teeth

The glad tidings are, you almost certainly shouldn't be. You can find three known reasons for that.

She'll outgrow it.

Most child industry experts agree that toddlers usually stop milling their teeth independently. They evidently just opt to stop one day and that's the end of it. It usually happens around age group six. At that time, they must be snoozing during the night with no milling or chomping.

How to proceed:

Go on and let them grind, but look out for any damage they could be triggering their tooth or gums. Check with your pediatrician if your child is milling his teeth at night age group of six.

It won't harm her teeth.

Among the reasons we don't want men and women to grind their tooth is that it might harm their tooth. Using a child, you don't need to be worried about that. It probably won't do any harm and if it can, those tooth are developing anyway.

If the tooth fairy has recently come and eliminated as well as your older child continues to be grinding away, speak to your child's dentist in regards to a tooth guard your child can wear during the night. The night time dam keeps tooth covered and can stop your son or daughter from milling their tooth. This usually isn't necessary until your child's long lasting tooth come in.

How to proceed:

Ask your child's dental practitioner to ensure there are no teeth fractures or other issues that could be leading to the milling. Ask if a night time dam may be beneficial.

The noise is the worst part.

Although your toddler's grinding could cause you some worry, it's good to learn that it's not really a serious condition, the noise you have to listen to is just about the worst type of part. So long as your baby doesn't appear to maintain pain and is sleeping during the night, you merely have to put on with the sound a little much longer.

How to proceed:

Make sure that your young child is sleeping peacefully and well regardless of the grinding.

What Never to Do

The worst thing you can certainly do with a toddler who's grinding their teeth is wake them up to prevent your child from grinding their teeth. Accomplishing this will frighten your son or daughter and hinder his ability to build up a regular sleep pattern.

Generally, trying to prevent your child from grinding their tooth is an awful idea for many reasons.

- ✓ They don't know they're carrying it out.
- ✓ Their known reasons for carrying it out aren't things they can control.
- ✓ If your child is milling his teeth because of anxiety, this will just make his anxiety worse.
- ✓ It isn't necessary. Teeth grinding probably isn't hurting your son or daughter.
- ✓ The Takeaway on Tooth Grinding

Your own worry is just about the worst part about learning that your child is grinding his teeth. The problem itself usually isn't serious, and it usually present once your son or daughter has completed teething. When you have concerns related to teeth damage, speak to your child's dental practitioner. If your young child is milling his tooth because of nervousness, speak to your child. With good luck and just a little tolerance, you can see through the milling and sleep sleepricted.

Chapter 21

Baby's Evening Light: Quarrels for & Against using Nightlights

Should My Baby Work with a Night Light?

The theory behind utilizing a baby night light is not strange because so many men and women are used to using night lighting. Sometimes, they think their baby may need one, too.

The answer will be there is nothing wrong with utilizing a baby night light, however, not using one is effective too. This may sound just a little complicated, but the pursuing points can help you understand why you might or might not want to employ a smooth light for your child at night.

Why do Parents Want the Light On?

There are multiple reasons why a parent should start the light for an infant; a few of these reasons are just misconceptions you have to recognize. Listed below are some reasons parents choose the light:

- ✓ You think getting the light can stop your child from getting scared, but infants don't fear whatever might be lurking at night.

- ✓ You imagine a night light will calm your child down, which is performed mainly for your satisfaction.

Now, this isn't to say a child won't ever get worried of what's lurking at night or won't feel less anxious with a light, but it won't happen when the kid is that small.

There are many reasons utilizing a baby night light may be beneficial, so you will learn about them:

Visual Development

Utilizing a baby evening light may help improve visual development. At this time, your infant is still changing to the light around her or him and is working quite hard.

Turning all the lighting off slows that process down, so

allowing your baby sleep with just a little light should power his/her eyes to keep working. Obviously, you can just allow moonlight flood directly into letting this happen normally, though this isn't always possible with respect to the position of your baby's room.

Sleepiness Boosted

Another justification a parent might be making the right decision when investing in a night light is basically because it might help your child sleep. As stated earlier, your child still can't see much, so she or he won't see those pretty baby mobiles rotating above the crib.

You will make it easier for your child to concentrate on those toys by utilizing a baby night light. Having the ability to see these playthings before drifting off to sleep helps an infant concentrate on a recurring sequence of occasions which should help your baby's brain feel less activated. You want this because an overstimulated brain is too alert, rendering it hard to fall or stay asleep.

Of course, you may be happy understanding that those

189

nightly baby checkups will be easier utilizing a baby evening light because you won't have to carefully turn on bright lighting that could wake your child up.

Why Should a Mother or Father Switch off the Light?

This decision won't be a simple one because there are two options for you. Still, it may be beneficial to recognize the myths there is no need to be concerned about, like the next:

✓ *Turning on the light in the night time could get your child used to sleeping with lamps on.*

✓ *Some parents think they want a light to see what's happening to their infants, but that's not true just because a baby will cry. Plus, some baby cams include nightvision.*

Now, there are a few genuine explanations why not utilizing a baby night time light might be considered a good notion for parents, like the next:

Learning Curve

Some experts say that infants can understand how to tell the difference between all the time. This is essential for the baby's overall knowledge of the world they're part of, but utilizing a baby night time light might hinder that important lesson.

Understand that area of the reason your child must learn the difference between all the time is because it can help inform the inner clock. The reason why you can awaken lacking any alarm is basically because you have a fairly good internal time clock.

You don't want your child to begin oversleeping because his/her internal clock is just a little off, right?

Sound Sleeping

There are a few experts who think that utilizing a baby night light will make it harder for an infant to sleep during the night. Associated with simply because the mind is learning that sunshine means melatonin shouldn't be produced.

Melatonin is a neurotransmitter which makes a person feel sleepy, and its own creation can be switched off by something similar to a night time light because the mind cannot show the difference between sunshine and artificial light.

You don't want to awaken in the center of the night time because your baby's brain was confused.

Conclusively; it is simple to see that we now have known reasons for utilizing a baby night time light and reasons to avoid artificial light. Obviously, your choice is eventually yours, but make an effort to consider both arguments prior to making a choice.

You might like to try both to observe how your baby reacts to both situations, and adhere to the one which is most effective. Do not interject your own emotions in to the decision; for example, don't start the light because you get worried of the dark. Keep in mind, babies are accustomed to sleeping in a pitch dark womb.

It could also be considered a good notion to speak to your

pediatrician concerning this decision because they might help you create an option. Take into account that the night time light situation could change as your child matures, so prepare yourself to turn from the light or switch the light on depending on your child's needs.

Chapter 22

The Bedtime Bottle: Breaking the Habit

Your child probably looks forward to his bottle at bedtime. As his mother or father, it could be hard to eliminate something he retains so dear, however the bedtime container can cause problems as your child ages. Weaning your child can result in a few evenings of tears and problems addressing sleep, but so long as it is performed in an adoring way, there is absolutely no reason behind it to cause much injury.

Between ages of six and nine or a few months, your child should be prepared to access sleep without a bottle at bedtime. By enough time he/she is a calendar year old, he/she really must quit the bottle. In the event that you wait a lot longer, the procedure becomes more challenging. Toddlers naturally develop very mounted on a regular, so waiting around until he/she is over twelve months old can make the procedure more difficult for you both.

You might wonder why it is so important to wean your

son or daughter from his bottle at bedtime. There are a number of reasons why utilizing a container to visit sleep is not really a good plan for you as well as your baby. Using the container creates a crutch in the bedtime regular. He'll have to eventually, and prolonging the procedure only allows him to develop more attached.

If you continue steadily to allow the container at bedtime following the age group where he needs it for nourishment, you might soon find that your child cannot drift off without a container in his mouth area.

One of the most practical reason you need to really get the bottle from your baby is that sucking on the bottle before he would go to sleep is bad for his recently emerging teeth.

Milk contains sugar that will adhere to one's teeth overnight, making a mating surface for the bacterias that can cause teeth decay. While dairy is bad, juice is a whole lot worse.

The first rung on the ladder in weaning your child is to

let him get accustomed to utilizing a cup. Many infants enjoy the chance to try consuming from a glass, even if it's a messy process to begin with. Once you are prepared to start out removing bottles, it seems sensible to begin with the container the child is least mounted on, which will probably not be his/her nighttime container.

Once your child is using a glass for his/her day time drinking, you will be ready to eliminate the container at bedtime. If he/she is a comparatively good eater, you will likely find that he/she will not even need the excess dairy at bedtime. Simply decrease the amount of dairy you give your child in the nighttime container a little every night; once your child is drinking simply a few ounces, offer drinking water rather than dairy in the glass.

You will likely think it is easiest to get all the bottles out of our home. This continues you from offering them up if either of you is experiencing a vulnerable moment. So long as he eats fairly well and has been presented to the glass, he doesn't require to have a container.

A bottle at bedtime will give a sense of comfort, which means you can introduce another form of comfort, like a stuffed animal early in the transitioning period. This enables him/her to get accustomed to utilizing it as his/her soother and won't view it as an alternative.

Why Get worried about Decay?

It may seem, baby tooth are temporary, why worry if indeed they create a little decay? Actually, decay in baby tooth can create huge issues. Due to small size of the infant tooth, they have less teeth enamel.

This makes them a lot more vunerable to decay than long lasting teeth. Decay in baby tooth must be treated, even although teeth are just temporary, otherwise, your son or daughter will experience oral pain and even early teeth loss.

Is there other issues with a bottle at bedtime?

Prolonged sucking on the bottle can cause issues with your child's oral development. The much longer your baby helps to keep the container in his mouth area, the much more likely it is to affect his bite. If your child is simply utilizing a container for milk several times a day, it isn't more likely to cause problems. If he uses it for relaxing, and retains it in his mouth area for longer intervals or falls asleep with it in his mouth area, he is more likely to develop oral issues.

While that may be scary, it's important to notice that turning to a glass can allow one's teeth to self-correct. Switching over from a container as quickly as possible minimizes the chances of your son or daughter developing issues from sucking on the container.

Another concern that can form from your son or daughter developing a bottle at bedtime are problems with diet. If your child is a good eater but insists on the nighttime milk container, he might gain more excess weight than is healthy.

On the contrary side of the problem, if your son or daughter is a picky eater, he might avoid trying new foods or eating foodstuffs that aren't his favorite because he understands he'll get a dairy container at bedtime. Small children only need about two mugs of milk each day, the others of their diet should consist of well balanced meals.

Methods to make the Container at Bedtime less Attractive

If your son or daughter is very mounted on his bottle, there are a few methods for you to make it less appealing.

✓ Drinking water down the milk

✓ Serve the dairy chilled, rather than warm

✓ Let her choose a glass she likes

✓ Let her help you to get her bedtime drink of drinking water within her nighttime routine

✓ Change the bedtime program to include cleaning teeth, snuggling, and cuddling a comfort object rather than going for a container to bed

Chapter 23

8 Ideas to Consider when Taking Baby to the Films

One of the primary problems that new moms face is to get out of the home with the youngster. Some won't even consider taking baby to the films because they dread it'll be a distraction to others. However, you don't have to be opening up in your own home because you have a child.

You can view those blockbuster movies rather than worry in regards to a sitter. Though baby's first-time at the cinema might now be considered a breeze, you will be ready to make sure they are comfortable and that means you can benefit from the show.

1 . Select a Movie that won't Startle the kid

When taking baby to the films, you will need to be sure you choose a film that won't startle them. Loud sounds, like gunshots or bombs, can simply put a child on advantage. If your son or daughter is screaming and crying throughout the complete show, you'll be seated outside rather than viewing the movie. You intend to ease them in to the movie theater experience by you starting with something that won't have a lot sound it causes their senses to get into overdrive.

You know your son or daughter much better than anyone. Baby's first-time at the cinema might not be a huge concern for you in any way. Some children could sleep through a hurricane and become unmoved. So use your very best judgment when choosing a film and choose something that is most beneficial for your child's sound comfort level.

2 . Choose Your Chairs Carefully

There are a huge selection of seats in the cinema, nevertheless, you want to be sure you choose your seat carefully. Never sit down in the centre where you'll need to crawl across ten visitors to get out to the sleeproom. Also, you don't want to sit down next to a couple of rowdy teenagers either, particularly if you may want to nurse.

The very best seats tend to be the ones in the trunk or the

ones neasleep to the entranceway. Remember, you can predict what sort of child will react, which means you desire to be ready for the unimaginable. Some up to date theaters have a particular place reserved for parents with small kids. They are usually close to the exits and also have boosters and other devices to help make the movie experience more enjoyable. Taking baby to the films is convenient when the theatre makes accommodations for parents.

3. Select a Less Packed and Cheaper Matinee Show

Because this outing is baby's first-time at the cinema, you might choose a less crowded matinee or daily teaching. First, they may be way less costly than night time shows, plus they frequently have a smaller audience.

You should attempt taking baby to the films if you are not paying a lot of money for tickets. If indeed they cannot sit down through the show, you'll be able to always leave understanding that you aren't out a couple of money.

4. Bring A lot of Dairy or Snacks

With regards to the age group of your son or daughter, you need a lot of food on their behalf. Taking baby to the films should never be achieved without snack foods and containers. A breastfed baby typically eats every two hours roughly. You will need to wear the right t-shirt for feeding in public areas.

If the kid is bottle given, then you want to be sure you have several containers on demand. The business from the home to the movie and back again can certainly be three or four hours in duration. If you don't want baby's first-time at the cinema to be filled up with food cravings and screaming out of hunger, then bring along nourishment.

5. Pack for the Unthinkable

Babies are recognized to proceed through several clothes per day. They are able to vomit, use the sleeproom and also have a variety of other issues. You will need to pack a huge handbag for baby's first-time at the cinema. You will include things such as spit up rags, moist wipes, diapers, playthings, and whatever might bring them comfort.

A couple of no specific things like bringing too much when taking baby to the films. Also, you might keep a supplementary clothing for you in the automobile just incase something happens.

6. Arrive Early

Taking baby to the films for the very first time is an experience. To avoid difficulties with locating the best chairs, and ensuring baby is given before the start of the show, make an effort to appear 15-20 minutes early. Baby's first-time at the cinema will be better if you come ready.

If you're going to a sold-out blockbuster, then you want to ensure that you allow the required time to enter and situated prior to the masses come. You can't just slide in with an infant and get the first chairs available. You will need time and careful planning.

7. Bring along Support Staff

If you wish to get any pleasure in any way from the show, you might want to bring along some support "personnel". Taking baby to the films with no help is a large undertaking.

If father cannot come, then you will want to bring grandma or a pal to help carry everything and help you should there be considered a meltdown at pivotal factors. You'll be thankful for the assistance if baby has a tough time at his first film show.

8. Use a Theatre that does Child Friendly Showings

If you're fortunate to have one particular theater that does kid-friendly showings, then it's a great spot to consider when taking baby to the films. Folks are also more understanding of these classes because they often have children too. Just how do they make the movie more child-friendly? They simply:

✓ Ignore the lamps for effect, however, not

completely change the lamps

- ✓ Lower the quantity of the movie to avoid scarring
- ✓ Shorten preview times to assist with brief attention spans

Remember these are heading to be "child friendly" G or PG-rated films. They aren't heading to provide these features with sold-out shows for the adult masses.

Taking Baby to the Movies

Don't avoid moving away from the house due to the fact you have a kid. You can figure out how to accommodate their needs but still have a great time for the time being. Remember, get one of these theatres that is accommodating to children and has shows where you will see lighter crowds. With some careful planning, you can view the greatest films but still have an infant in tow.

Chapter 24

Levels of Crawling and Rolling Over: Baby Timeline

Infants reach developmental milestones at different age groups, and getting those milestones at a youthful or later age group than most is definitely not a reason for alarm.

If your son or daughter is constantly achieving milestones later than her peers, it seems sensible to go over your concerns with your pediatrician. Although there's a wide range in what's considered healthy, it is normal to question, "when will my baby crawl?" or "when will my baby move over?"

Developmental milestones vary among babies, however in general, in your baby's first year you may expect her to:

✓ Roll from entrance to back

✓ Roll from back to front

✓ Sit supported

- ✓ Sit independently

- ✓ Crawl

- ✓ Assume a seated position without help

- ✓ Move between positions independently (sitting down, crawling, laying on tummy)

- ✓ Draw into a stand

- ✓ Cruise (walk, keeping furniture or a grown-up)

- ✓ Move a ball

- ✓ Have a few unassisted steps

When Will My Baby Move Over?

There are a few things your child needs to have the ability to do before he/she actually is prepared to roll over. Your child will move over when he/she is in control over her mind.

Rolling over typically builds up once your baby begins seated up with support. Your child will move over from her tummy to her back again first generally. Offering a lot of tummy time is a superb way to encourage moving over.

Once your child can move from tummy to back again, and again, she'll quickly learn she can maneuver around just a little this way. This is actually the beginning to become mobile, which is more important than ever before to monitor her. Soon, your child will move over as a strategy to reach her favorite toy, or even to you.

Your baby will most likely start endeavoring to kick over onto her back again from her tummy at around four months old. Some babies grab this skill quickly, while some have a while. Once your child can move over from tummy to back again it will require somewhat much longer to turn from back again to tummy.

Flipping onto the belly from the trunk uses more coordination and neck of the guitar and equip strength than flipping from the belly to back again. Once she can move from her tummy to back, your child will move over from back again to front within a couple weeks.

Your child will move over when she develops the power

and coordination essential to perform the maneuver. You are able to help her out by offering a lot of supervised tummy time. While laying on the tummy, your baby begins raising his/her chest muscles up with his/her hands at around three months.

This is actually the beginning of building the strength needed to flip over. Generally, by enough time your child is six months old, he/she will have the ability to move both from his/her tummy to back again and from back again to tummy.

When Will My Baby Crawl?

Your child will crawl once and developed the power and coordination essential to balance on hands and knees. For some infants, this is between age range of seven and ten a few months. It's important to notice that not absolutely all infants crawl in a normal manner.

Some get right up on the hands and knees and rock and roll backwards and forwards, eventually continue in a normal crawl, while some scoot on the bottom while in a sitting down position, army crawl using their elbows, or even maneuver around by rolling. Some infants skip crawling completely and begin by tugging themselves through to furniture and cruising along.

So long as your child is advancing and determining how to be mobile, your child will crawl when he/she actually is ready and his/her form will not matter.

Your child will crawl within a natural development from understanding how to move over and sit without having to be supported. You will find actions you can take to help your child expert these skills. As with moving over, tummy time is important. Tummy time helps your child develop the power and coordination needed to support his/herself.

Putting some special toys and games on the floor, just away from baby's reach, during tummy time can be all the encouragement your child needs to become mobile.

Must I Worry?

It really is normal for new parents to question, when will my baby move over? When will my baby crawl? Understand that these quantities are just suggestions. If your son or daughter was premature, your child will crawl and reach other milestones nearer to what her age group would be if she were full-term.

Personality also offers too much to do with these milestones. An infant with a quiet, laidback character may become more content to place quietly watching activity while an infant with a far more energetic or challenging personality could be more willing to squirm, fuss and generally maneuver around in a manner that builds up the power and coordination essential to move.

It is worthy of note that not absolutely all babies take part in all milestones. For instance, some infants never crawl, after they learn how to take a seat on their own, they quickly draw themselves up and make an effort to get good at walking. It isn't necessary that your son or daughter performs each milestone, but she should be, continue and look, thinking about learning new skills.

What goes on if my Child will not Roll over or Crawl promptly?

It's important to notice that your child will crawl, move over and walk independently on timeframe. These skills are just one single part of your baby's development. These activities are known as gross electric motor skills. There's also fine electric motor skills, such as grasping items, vocabulary and communication skills, and public skills.

Your son or daughter may be advanced in a single expertise but lag behind in another. So long as she actually is making ahead progress, it isn't generally a reason for concern.

If your son or daughter does not appear to be making improvement in a single area, such as his/her gross engine skills, or appears to lag in a number of areas, you should speak to your pediatrician about your concerns.

Most likely your son or daughter will meet up with his/her peers by enough time he/she begins college, but early treatment is very beneficial regarding developmental delays.

Chapter 25

7 Signs or symptoms Your Child is Lactose Intolerant

When you have a problem that your child may be lactose intolerant, it is most likely because you have observed something about your child or their toileting conditions that has you concerned. You might suspect that your child is lactose intolerant, but want to determine if indeed they are actually. Below, we've even more information that will help you see whether your child truly comes with an intolerance towards lactose.

What is Lactose?

Lactose is the sugars that is situated in milk. It really is within cow's dairy as well as breastmilk. Additionally, most formulas are dairy-based and also contain lactose.

What does it mean to become Lactose Intolerant?

If one is lactose intolerant, this means that their body struggles to break the lactose down enough such that it is simple to digest. Our anatomies produce lactase, a digestive enzyme, which works inside our gut to breakdown the lactose. If a person or baby is lactose intolerant, this means that their body isn't in a position to produce enough lactase to sufficiently break down the lactose. This may lead to the individual or baby experiencing unpleasant side effects.

If your child is lactose intolerant, it generally does not mean they have a dairy allergy. Having a lactose intolerance, the person's body isn't in a position to properly breakdown the lactose; with a dairy allergy, they may be allergic and respond to the protein in the dairy.

A dairy allergy is normally more serious than lactose intolerant. You can find three types of lactose intolerances below:

Major: This form of lactose intolerant typically doesn't develop until later in one's life. This sort of intolerance may appear because of the body ingesting less lactose than it is normally used to. This may also happen in people or cultures that don't eat many products comprising lactose.

Secondary: That is typically a short-term form of lactose intolerance. It could sometimes be triggered by contamination, disease, or antibiotics that are used for a long period of time.

Congenital: If your child is lactose intolerant, chances are the congenital form of intolerance. With this hereditary form of the intolerance, infants are not given birth to with sufficient levels of lactase to split up the lactose in dairy.

Some premature babies are also given birth to with lactose intolerance because of the fact that their small intestine is not developed enough. In the majority of these situations, the infants outgrow their lactose intolerance with time.

Signs that your Child could be Lactose Intolerant

If you think that your child may be lactose intolerant, there are many signs or symptoms you can look for to help you select. A pediatrician can continually be a great reference if you want to determine if your child is lactose intolerant.

Crying Frequently

Whenever a baby is lactose intolerant, they are generally uncomfortable. Their physiques can't breakdown the lactose, which is hard on the little physiques. This will most likely cause your child to cry more often as they express their soreness.

Diarrhea

When your body can't properly breakdown the lactose

within milk, it could lead to diarrhea. If you notice a great deal of diarrhea, it could be an indicator that your child is lactose intolerant.

Vomiting

Again, the shortcoming for your body to properly break down and break down the lactose can result in vomiting. When your body can't properly process something, it sometimes comes home up by means of vomit.

Gas or Loud Colon Sounds

If your child is lactose intolerant, you may observe that they have a lot of gas of make loud sounds because they are pooping.

Green or Yellow Stools

In babies, lactose intolerance can frequently change just how their stools look. In the event that you notice watery green or yellowish stools, it could mean that your child is lactose intolerant.

Poor Putting on Weight

Sometimes whenever a baby has a lactose intolerance they don't gain enough weight. Because the lactose intolerance can cause throwing up and diarrhea, this may sometimes donate to poor putting on weight in an infant.

Pores and skin Rashes or Recurring Colds

Lactose intolerance can also sometimes lead to rashes on your skin or regular colds. So, if you have observed either of the symptoms in your child, it might be a sign they are lactose intolerant.

Will my Child be Lactose Intolerant Forever?

It's possible that your child might not be lactose intolerant later in their life. If your child being given birth to prematurely was the reason with regards to lactose intolerance, then it's possible that they could outgrow the intolerance later in life as their small intestine proceeds to develop.

When you talk to your pediatrician, they can talk about their thoughts about whether your child may outgrow their lactose intolerance.

What must I do Suspecting that my Baby is Lactose Intolerant?

If you think that your child has a lactose intolerance, there are many different steps you should immediately try help alleviate their symptoms.

Speak to your Pediatrician

Your first call ought to be to your baby's pediatrician. They'll be in a position to help you see whether your child will indeed have a lactose intolerance.

When you are through, the indications which may have resulted in you thinking of the intolerance, the pediatrician will help you determine if indeed they point to your child being lactose intolerant or if indeed they may be triggered by another issue that requires attention.

Change their Diet

If your child is lactose intolerant, you're going to have to change their diet. If they're formula-fed, there are lactose-free formulas you can change to.

Your pediatrician can also help you decide on the best type or make of formula for your child.

If you're breastfeeding, your pediatrician may recommend using lactase drops. These drops can help your baby break down the lactose in your breastmilk.

Avoid Food which contain Lactose

If your child has already been eating food, or after they become old enough to start eating solids, you'll want to be certain to avoid feeding them foods which contain lactose. Also, be certain to check on labels on any prepackaged foods, as much foods contain substances with lactose.

It could be worrisome if you believe your child is lactose intolerant. But, once you utilize the signs or symptoms to recognize the lactose intolerance, with simply a few adjustments, your child can continue steadily to grow and prosper!

Chapter 26

My Baby Isn't Growing! What MAY I Do?

Expecting can be an exhausting but exhilarating experience. Once you've given birth compared to that small creature, your priorities immediately change. You are abruptly consumed with looking after your brand-new baby. You intend to see them healthy, growing, and flourishing.

It could be very concerning if you learn that your child isn't growing. As a fresh mother or father, it's possible you're feeling just like a failure and it's sure that you'll wish to accomplish all you can to really get your baby back again on the right track and attaining weight.

If you're concerned about your brand-new baby's putting on weight, read below for a few tips to help you see whether there happens to be a problem and for a few recommendations for how to help your child get healthier and put on weight. It's also a good idea to get in touch with your child's pediatrician if you are worried about their putting on weight.

What's Normal?

It's important to find out that each baby grows and develops differently. Because your child isn't getting as much weight as other infants you understand, isn't necessarily grounds to get worried. Also, many infants lose weight of their first couple of days of life, and then need to get it back again to make contact with their delivery weight. Below are a few typical milestones most healthy, growing infants meet. But, again, understand that every baby differs.

- ✓ Most pediatricians prefer to visit a baby back at their delivery weight within two to ten weeks after delivery.

- ✓ Most healthy babies increase their labor and birth weight by enough time they are half a year.

- ✓ Most healthy babies triple their labor and birth weight by enough time are twelve months old.

If your child isn't conference their growth and putting on weight milestones, they might be labeled with failure to thrive.

This name definitely sounds worrisome. Many parents who have a baby who's labeled with failing to thrive are rightfully very worried. But, you'll find so many tips and strategies you can test to make if your child isn't growing and getting enough weight.

Why isn't my Baby Adding Weight? What Should I do

There are many reasons why your child isn't growing and gaining enough weight. Again, every baby differs, so you'll should do some work, observations, and conversations with medical staff to look for the exact reason your child isn't growing and getting weight.

Here are some possible causes that you can investigate and consult with a pediatrician or lactation specialist to help you pinpoint the reason why your child isn't growing. Below are possible causes for insufficient putting on weight; we've offered you some recommendations for what you can test to help if you believe that's the reason your child isn't growing.

Your Child isn't Eating Enough From Each Feeding

A reason your child isn't growing could be because of the fact that they aren't getting enough dairy from each feeding. If you're breastfeeding, this may imply that they aren't remaining latched on long enough to transfer enough dairy. It might also be a sign that you will find a low way to obtain dairy and aren't producing enough dairy to provide them sufficient calorie consumption during the day. If your child isn't bottle-fed, you might not be offering them enough at each nourishing.

What may I do to help my Baby?

If you're worried that your child isn't getting enough dairy at each feeding, there are many things you can test. First, consult with your pediatrician about the quantity of food your child should be getting each day, and separate that by the amount of times your child is eating every day. This will give you a concept of how much dairy your child should be getting from each nourishing.

Typically, pediatricians advise that your child be fed between two and three ounces of milk for every pound they weigh (however, not to exceed thirty-two ounces of milk per day). So, if your child weighs six pounds, they need to eat between twelve and eighteen ounces per day. If your child weight eight pounds, they need to eat between sixteen and twenty-four ounces per day. Most pediatricians advise that your child gets between twenty-four and thirty-two ounces of milk per day after they are a couple of months old.

If you're worried that low breastmilk source may be the reason why your child isn't getting enough dairy, first utilize a lactation advisor to execute a weighted give food to. They are able to weigh your child before and after a breastfeeding program to observe how much dairy they were in a position to transfer.

If it doesn't appear to be they are receiving enough dairy, there will vary things you can test to boost your dairy supply. You can find supplements that can help increase dairy production. Additionally, searching online for a few lactation cookie dishes that are created with things that can result in more dairy being produced.

If your child isn't getting enough dairy from each feeding and you are breastfeeding, you may want to consider supplementing with some formula. You want to ensure that your child gets enough dairy to be healthy. Once it is possible to up your dairy supply, you might be able to scale back on the quantity of formula your child gets every day if you would like to attempt to exclusively breastfeed.

You Aren't Feeding Your child Frequently Enough

In the event that you aren't feeding your child enough times throughout the day, this may also donate to your child not gaining enough weight. Infants, especially newborns, employ a tiny abdomen and can only just hold a small amount of milk at the same time. So, they have to eat very frequently, especially during those first couple of days and weeks of their lives.

What may I do to help my Baby?

Again, understand that an infant needs somewhere within two and three ounces of dairy for every pound they weigh each day. If you've noticed that your child isn't achieving this total by the finish of your day, you'll want to raise the number of that time period you a nourishing her or him.

Many newborn and incredibly young babies need to consume every two hours, often at night time as well. Once your child is just a little old and their abdomen can take more at each nourishing, you might be able to pass on feedings out a little more. Soon, your child might be able to get enough dairy throughout the day to have the ability to sleep during the night, or at least sleep for an extended stretch out. But, again, every baby differs, and some might need to continue the night time feedings for much longer than others.

Your Child isn't Latching to Your Breasts Well

If your child isn't obtaining a good latch on your breast, they might not be transferring enough dairy, even if it seems these are nursing for a long period. A tongue or lip connect is actually a possible reason your child isn't in a position to latch to your breast.

What may I do to greatly help my Baby?

If you're uncertain if your child has a good, efficient latch, a very important thing to do is to seek advice from a lactation expert. They are able to observe your infants latch and present you tips about how to achieve a much better latch which means that your baby gets enough dairy. As stated above, a lactation expert can also execute a weighted give food to your child to observe how much dairy are actually moving from each program.

If you believe your baby's poor latch may be due to a tongue or lip link, a pediatrician or lactation expert can test your baby's mouth area to determine when there is a concern. If your child has a tongue or lip connect, it's important to obtain it fixed once you can to help them enhance their latch. The procedure for repairing a tongue or lip connect is not at all hard and quick. It will require your baby a while to re-learn how to nurse after getting the process done, so don't expect an instantaneous change in their latch and medical.

Your Baby has a Food Intolerance or Allergy

A reason your child isn't growing could be because they come with an allergy or intolerance to dairy. Some infants have a milk protein intolerance, this means their body can't absorb the protein from milk, that could lead to them not attaining enough weight.

What may I do to help my Baby?

If you think that a dairy intolerance may be the reason

your child isn't growing, definitely get hold of your pediatrician. They are able to ask you more specific questions to help see whether an intolerance is to be blamed for your child not attaining enough weight. Your pediatrician can also send you for an allergist if indeed they suspect there's a food allergy.

A Sickness or other Condition is causing loss of weight

It's possible that a disease or underlying condition may be the cause why your child is not gaining enough weight. Some possible conditions that may be adding to why your child isn't growing include acid reflux disorder, chronic diarrhea, celiac disease, metabolic disorders, or issues with your baby's center or lungs.

What may I do to help my Baby?

You should see your child if you suspect anything is wrong with them. Make sure to match the regular pediatric visits through the first season of their life. Vaccinating your son or daughter following the suggested CDC plan is also important to stop your baby becoming unwell.

It could be very concerning whenever your baby isn't growing and gaining weight. You are normally very concerned because of their health insurance and wish to accomplish whatever you can to help them thrive.

Hopefully the suggestions and recommendations we offered in this specific article can help you determine the reason for your baby's poor putting on weight and find a remedy for the problem. Pediatricians and lactation consultants may also be excellent resources to help get your child on the right course towards reaching a wholesome weight and growing!

Chapter 27

Why Giving Your Child Water is more Threatening than You Imagine

If you're a mother or father or a soon-to-be-mother or father, it's likely that sooner or later you're going to be paranoid about everything, including something less than giving your child water. Works out your concerns aren't unfounded, because to put it simply, if you're questioning: 'can I give my baby drinking water?', 'could it be safe?', the answer is *No*.

No Drinking Water for Six Months

When you want to keep your child hydrated, in most cases, giving your child water is a huge no-no until your child is about six months old.

Until that age group, they get all the required hydration from formula or breasts milk, irrespective of weather. Dehydration is an ailment that needs to be taken seriously, and if you believe that your child is not getting enough liquid, then it's time to get hold of your doctor.

You can merely tell if they're hydrated enough by counting the wet diapers. Until they may be six months old, they must have at least six damp diapers every day.

Indicators of dehydration that you can look include having fewer bowel motions, being excessively sleepy or fussy, cool discolored feets and hands, wrinkled pores and skin, or sunken eye. In some instances, if the infant has belly flu, for example, your physician might advise that you provide them with Infalyte or Pedialyte, or other electrolyte drink to keep them from becoming dehydrated.

Why is Giving Your child Water Dangerous?

Until they may be six months old, the kidneys of the infant aren't mature enough to filtering water correctly, thus leaving them vunerable to water intoxication.

Even when they may be six months old, if an infant beverages too much drinking water, it can hinder the power that his body must absorb the nutritional vitamins from formula or breasts milk. Furthermore, the child's abdomen will feel full and he/she would not want to consume anymore.

In a few rare instances, babies who drink too much water can finish up developing what's known as water intoxication, that could lead to seizures or perhaps a coma. This happens when the focus of sodium in their person is diluted by too much drinking water, thus creating cells to swell consequently of upsetting the electrolyte balance.

Sip by Sip

After they are six months old, offering your baby drinking water in smaller amounts is safe, and never have to be concerned about any issues. It really is ideal though to only offer little items of drinking water at the same time, as they don't require it just as much as grown-ups, and drinking water won't replace method or breast dairy, which is essential for the first twelve months of their life.

Until they may be a year old, giving your child water should be observed only as practice, and therefore you can provide them a few sips once in a while, as infants also get accustomed to the sippy glass around that point. The theory is to get the tiny one familiar to normal water. After they are nine to a year old, they can drink a few ounce of drinking water every day.

Diluting Formula with Water. Is it safe?

If you increase much drinking water, not only does it increase the chance of drinking water intoxication, however the baby might finish up getting fewer nutrition from the formula. Furthermore, too much drinking water could screw up their electrolyte balance. To avoid problems, simply adhere to the suggestions, or use breasts milk instead. When coming up with method, you should follow the directions on the bundle and use the quantity of water that is preferred.

Bonus: Taking in Juice?

Giving your child water once they are six months old is

the healthiest choice, and can have them used to it. Alternatively, it is ideal that drinking water is the only drink that you present, as there is absolutely no rush. Regarding to pediatrician Catherine Pound, Juice is absolutely not essential, and it's simply glucose. She advises that if parents will provide them with juice, they need to ensure that it's real juice, plus they should offer only 4oz/day.

In conclusion, the next time you consider, 'can I give my baby water?', make an effort to keep this at heart:

- ✓ Giving your child drinking water is unsafe until they are in least six months old
- ✓ Smaller amount of water is enough
- ✓ Diluting formula with too much drinking water is dangerous
- ✓ Giving your child water won't replace formula/breasts milk.

Chapter 28

Almond Dairy: Is it Safe for Your Child?

Almond dairy is great tasting low calorie drink that people and children can enjoy.

What's there never to love in regards to a beverage created from almonds and drinking water?

Still, could it be safe for your child?

The short answer is *NO*, not if your child is under one. The long answer is nutritional density in comparison with other options still doesn't supply the nutrition your child or children require.

Issues that could occur with offering your child almond dairy before their first birthday:

- ✓ Breastfeeding issues, such as refusal to latch

- ✓ Vitamin and nutrient deficiency

- ✓ Failing to grow or put on weight

- ✓ Refusal to consume.

May I Give my Baby Almond Dairy at

Treat Time?

Pediatricians often make reference to turning or weaning from formulation or breast dairy to almond dairy. Giving your child almond dairy at treat time shouldn't result in a problem unless your child comes with an allergy or you're still solely breastfeeding.

Before giving your child almond milk or other beverages, you should seek advice from with pediatrician. Take into account that your baby's doctor might help you to hold back if your loved ones have a brief history of tree nut allergy symptoms.

In some instances, she or he might supply the green light for almond milk as a treat time beverage. However, don't present almond milk prior to the age of one without their go-ahead.

You Suspect Your Child has a Dairy Allergy and want to try Almond Milk

Dairy allergies and intolerances are normal, but giving your child almond dairy isn't the answer. Allergy and intolerance symptoms may differ, but gas, cramping, constipation, and diarrhea may appear with intolerance. Rashes, hives, and bloating can also happen.

It's important to go over these symptoms as well as your concerns with your pediatrician before providing your child almond dairy. If your child shows indications of facial bloating or bloodstream in their stools, you should call your physician immediately.

For milder symptoms, your physician might prefer to perform tests or start an eradication diet. Breast nourishing mothers will also embark on a special diet because the foods and beverages they consume move into their dairy. Once you as well as your pediatrician find the reason, they'll recommend an effective treatment that will be of advantage to your baby's ever growing needs.

In some instances, what you suspected as a dairy allergy could grow to be something else. Your child could have multiple food allergy symptoms or intolerances too. Providing your child almond milk will make locating the cause harder too if your child has a response. Food and drink could be unrelated to your child's symptoms. It's important never to attempt analysis by yourself.

Almond Dairy Safe For Teenagers and Toddlers?

Almond Dairy is an excellent choice for adults, and maybe it's for your teenagers too. Giving your child almond milk older than one might still need you to product with other food stuffs or vitamins. Make sure to ask your physician.

Missing Nutrition, Vitamins, and Minerals from Almond Milk

Breast dairy or formula will be the best selections for your baby because they support the nutrition your growing baby needs. Commercial almond milks might be fortified, but homemade types plus some brands still absence many essential minerals and vitamins.

Take into account that the same pertains to other plant-based dairy alternatives. Their meals address the needs of adults. Plant-based milks and drinks are not add up to formulation, breast dairy, or cow's dairy in conditions of the nutrition. Some doctors still recommend additional supplements for children more than a calendar year old and to their teenagers because the fortified drinks still flunk.

Switching your child to almond dairy too early will rob them of key nutrition that plant-based milks can't contend with. It does not have the fat molecules, including saturated fats your baby's body and systems need to operate and develop. Almond dairy also doesn't contain brain healthy essential fatty acids like DHA and ALA.

Proteins can be another area where your child won't receive what they want. Breast dairy and baby formulas contain multiple proteins chains that your child easily digests. Plant-based formulas will imitate this to ensure they offer your child with an entire protein string too. Giving your son or daughter almond dairy can cause tummy annoyed because plant-based dairy beverages don't support the soft proteins your child can digest.

Other Concerns about Offering Your Child Almond Milk

If you've ever walked down the dairy products aisle, you've witnessed firsthand just how many brands and types of almond dairy exist. Most of them contain added things that your child doesn't need. These substances range between added sugar and tastes to thickeners and preservatives.

Exercise caution and limit these varieties of almond milk.

If your child has ended a year old or you have your pediatrician's permission, opt for unsweetened, unflavored almond dairy.

Chapter 29

Giving Your Child Yogurt: Could it be Safe?

Giving your child yogurt is definitely a thrilling experience, as they move from formula/breasts milk to solids. You almost certainly thought about; 'can I give my baby yogurt?', and it changes that it's a safe choice. Generally, infants can begin eating yogurt when they could eat solids.

You should seek advice from your doctor upon this matter if you would like to be sure; many doctors have been recommending that you introduce yogurt when your child is nine to ten a few months old. Alternatively, recent studies led some pediatrics to advise that you start offering your child yogurt (some types from it, such as dairy or ordinary) as soon as six months.

Great Things about giving Your Child Yogurt

Yogurt is effective and nutritional to infants who are six months and older. Yogurt is a convenient way to obtain protein, and they have less lactose compare to dairy;

246

babies can withhold the enzyme to be able to breakdown lactose.

The existence of probiotics in yogurts is also important. Yogurt can fine melody the disease fighting capability which lines the intestine, thus assisting the body of your infant understand which bacterias is dangerous and which is effective.

Lactose Intolerance? Could it be safe?

It is well worth noting however that giving your child yogurt can lead to an allergic attack in those who have dairy allergies. They are able to take place in around 2-3% of newborns, symptoms including vomiting, diarrhea, epidermis rashes, bloating, and irritability.

Much like any new food that you introduce, you should wait around at least three times before you introduce a fresh one. That way, in case there is an allergic attack you can pin point the reason. As observed, lactose intolerance is very uncommon among infants, and even if the infant might become lactose intolerant, it might be safe to allow them to eat yogurt, as it is easier tolerated in comparison to other milk products.

If indeed they show symptoms of a food allergy, or has been identified as having a dairy allergy, speak to your doctor before you select giving your child yogurt.

Why is Giving Your Child Yogurt Okay?

The medical community advises against dairy products before a baby is twelve months old, as they worry that if parents introduce Whole Cow dairy, they might stop using formula or breastfeeding and use dairy as an alternative. Replacing method/breast dairy with Entire Cow dairy is dangerous to the fitness of the baby.

Alternatively, giving your child yogurt (and cheese for example) will not put the infant in danger, and therefore parents won't replace formula with yogurt. Lactose gets divided with the culturing of the yogurt, and the dairy proteins are limited or semi-removed. Furthermore, the culturing makes yogurt easy to break down.

Types of Yogurt

It's ideal to be selective when selecting yogurt for you baby. There are many choices on the marketplace that are tagged for kids, nevertheless, you should still focus on what you're buying. Be sure you select a dairy yogurt, because of the fact that the infant needs the healthy fat that is within the yogurt to be able to build up properly. Furthermore, while all yogurt has normally occurring sugars, be sure you know about how much glucose it includes and if it offers other chemicals, such as starches, fructose syrup, etc .

You could start with plain, dairy yogurt, and to be able to include flavor you can stir in a veggie of fruit purée that your child might tolerate. Being an aspect note: accomplishing this will also finish up helping you save money, as yogurt advertised for infants are more costly as well.

May I Give my Baby Yogurt? Could it be safe?

When you see giving your child yogurt, retain in mind the next:

- ✓ Yogurt is a safe choice after the baby is needed to eat solids

- ✓ If your child is lactose intolerant, they could still be in a position to eat yogurt - check along with your doctor to be sure.

- ✓ Focus on extra sugar in the yogurt you select - a perfect choice is to go with natural yogurt

- ✓ Dairy products aren't recommended for infants until they are at least twelve months old, but eating yogurt and cheese are alright.

Chapter 30

Strange Child Sleeping Habits Explained
Strange Sleeping Practices of Children

Among the joys of parenting is that calm moment during the night when you try looking in at the sleeping child. In the dim light, she actually is so relaxed, peaceful and beautiful; yet many children develop unusual sleeping practices. Sometimes these practices are a stage, and sometimes they could point to a far more serious concern. Read on to comprehend some of unusual sleeping practices of children.

Baby Only Sleeps with a Light On

Many parents express concern in regards to a child who only sleeps with the lighting on. This isn't discussing your standard, dim nightlight, but only drifting off to sleep when the over head light is on. For parents, a kid who sleeps with a light on is stressing since there is not really a normal changeover from day time to sleep time. Most of all, lights in the area can disrupt a child's normal sleep patterns.

Baby is Afraid of the Dark

The natural rhythm for humans is usually to be awake throughout the day and asleep during the night. Evening vision is much less good as day eyesight, so things simply look different during the night. Many children proceed through a stage of being scared of the dark. Most children are content with a little nightlight, however, many want a brighter source to feel safe.

Baby is Afraid of Drifting Off to Sleep

If you believe about it, sleep is a strange event. You close your eye and lose eight hours. For a few children, that idea can be terrifying. There may be worries that something might eventually occur to the kid while he/she sleeping. There may be worries of passing up on intesleeping things during sleep. Keeping the lighting on becomes a technique for keeping sleep at bay.

A Parent's Response

For some children, both these anxieties represent a passing stage. If indeed they last too much time, you might talk to a specialist psychologist for help. Some parents think it is beneficial to wean children from light resources, using lower wattage lights in the over head fixture until it could be turned off completely. The kid still sleeps with a light on, but it becomes gradually dimmer.

Baby Sleeps with Face Under a Pillow

You peek in your son or daughter's bedroom where he/she should be fast asleep, nevertheless, you do not see his/her adorable face. Looking nearer, you find that your child has face under a cushion. Why on the planet would your child do this?

It makes him/her feel secure

Some children express a concern with the night time by using blankets and pillows as a cocoon of safety. The connection with the smooth areas offers them warmness and comfort. In cases like this, whenever your child sleeps with his/her mind under a cushion, it is merely an effort to feel a bit more secure during the night.

It blocks out noise

If your son or daughter has trouble drifting off to sleep, he/she may but put his/her head under the pillow since it blocks out sound or other types of stimulation. For instance, a kid whose room encounters a busy road might cover her check out block out road sounds and the lamps from headlights that go by.

A Parent's response

This behavior is also normally a phase. As the kid grows older, she'll be less reliant on cushions and blankets for comfort. So long as she actually is sleeping easily, you can leave it only. If it's a matter of excitement, blackout tones can stop outside sound and lamps. If your son or daughter struggles to offer with outside excitement at all, you might have him/her examined by your physician.

Baby Sleeps with Mouth Open

A common problem for both people and children is sleeping using their mouths open. Mouth-breathing during the night can result in snoring and drooling throughout sleep and bad breathing each day. In the long run, this habit in children can also lead to teeth milling and orthodontic issues as well as sleep deprivation.

A Mouth-Breathing Habit

It isn't unusual for children who breathe through their mouths throughout the day to do the same when they sleep. Mouth-breathing could just be a stage, where your son or daughter is tinkering with how respiration feels. However, it could also indicate some medical conditions that should be examined.

A Medical Condition

There are many medical ailments that lead to sleeping with the mouth open. Most has to do with the anatomy of the child's mind and throat, conditions that produce respiration through the nasal area difficult. They include:

- ✓ Deviated septum

- ✓ Enlarged tonsils

- ✓ Enlarged adenoids

- ✓ Allergies or an infection with nose congestion.

A Parent's response

If your son or daughter has a cold or seasonal allergies, mouth-breathing will pass when the symptoms get rid of. If your son or daughter always sleeps along with his mouth area open, seek advice from your pediatrician to see when there is an root condition.

Baby Sticks Tongue away at Night

You take a look at your son or daughter sleeping during

intercourse and he/she sticks her tongue out at you. It really is a foolish face, but for anyone who is worried? Sleeping with her tongue out is another uncommon sleeping habit.

Area of the Latching Reflex

The tongue-thrust reflex is area of the latching process children use when these are breastfeeding. If your son or daughter continues to be breastfeeding or has stopped, protruding her tongue may simply be an unconscious action. She may be fantasizing about nourishing, or this might just happen when she swallows in her sleep.

A Physical Issue

Whenever your child sleeps with her tongue away, it could be a sign of the physical issue. She may come with an enlarged tongue or a particularly small mouth area. These conditions will probably be your child's hereditary luck-of-the-draw, however they may also be indications of much more serious hereditary conditions that should be analyzed.

A Parent's Response

Protruding her tongue when she sleeps is most likely something your son or daughter will outgrow. Each young one develops in a different way; some may store the latching reflex much longer than others. If this is a matter of the scale, have your child's tongue or mouth area analyzed within a routine health and fitness.

Lightning Source UK Ltd.
Milton Keynes UK
UKHW021221161220
375273UK00008B/525